HYPNOTISM

The Practical Introduction to Therapeutic
Hypnosis

(Learn How to Manipulate Others and Make
Them Do Your Bidding)

Shelley Walls

Published by Ryan Princeton

Shelley Walls

All Rights Reserved

Hypnotism: The Practical Introduction to Therapeutic Hypnosis (Learn How to Manipulate Others and Make Them Do Your Bidding)

ISBN 978-1-77485-338-2

Legal & Disclaimer

The information contained in this book is not designed to replace or take the place of any form of medicine or professional medical advice. The information in this book has been provided for educational and entertainment purposes only.

The information contained in this book has been compiled from sources deemed reliable, and it is accurate to the best of the Author's knowledge; however, the Author cannot guarantee its accuracy and validity and cannot be held liable for any errors or omissions. Changes are periodically made to this book. You must consult your doctor or get professional medical advice before using any of the suggested remedies, techniques, or information in this book.

Upon using the information contained in this book, you agree to hold harmless the Author from and against any damages, costs, and expenses, including any legal fees potentially resulting from the application of any of the information provided by this guide. This disclaimer applies to any damages or injury caused by the use and application, whether directly or indirectly, of any advice or information presented, whether for breach of contract, tort, negligence, personal injury, criminal intent, or under any other cause of action.

You agree to accept all risks of using the information presented inside this book. You need to consult a professional medical practitioner in order to ensure you are both able and healthy enough to participate in this program.

Table of Contents

Introduction

In these pages, you're going to be taught everything you'll need before you can begin using hypnosis to aid in therapeutic and entertainment purposes.

This isn't a massive book of theory but it is a plan, this book is about hypnosis in the practice. Its counterpart, will provide hypnosis practical and theoretical and will attempt to create the complete curriculum and an essential desk reference as well as a field guide.

At first, you'll want apply your skills to your family and friends. I strongly recommend doing this. It is learned through experience and hypnosis is no exception practicing makes perfect. So learn from this book the techniques and then apply these techniques.

In terms of the theory, you don't need much knowledge to be able to use hypnosis effectively, it is important to understand that it is a natural process, we fall into trance whenever you tie your shoes or pick up the phone or give in the preconditioned response to an event such as a situation, state or event.

We can be amazed or shocked. We enter trance to attempt to understand what went wrong.

Hypnosis with some name or another has been around since Egypt but it became more popular in the 21st century with Mesmer, Braid and Elman. A little bit of research can give you lots of details about people who were hypnotists and their influence on the art of. Hypnosis is used for therapeutic purposes to aid in faster healing as well as anaesthetic and pain management as well as to release previously suppressed memories, curing fears and much more.

Chapter 1: Hypnosis: Myth & Realitycan slide from one state to the next quite easily.

Hypnosis Myth & Reality

Hollywood hype will make us believe that hypnotists are able to influence and control your actions and it is possible to do unbelievable things when hypnotized. Here are a few of the most common myths which need to be cleared before proceeding.

The hypnotist could force you to commit actions against your wishes.

Absolutely false. The hypnotist does not have any power over you in any way and cannot force you to take actions against your wishes. Everything about Hypnosis is truly self-directed and self-controlled. The hypnotist simply leads you into the state of hypnosis, and then feeds your brain by providing carefully worded suggestions. If you are uncomfortable with the suggestions, you are free to choose to ignore them. Hypnosis is in essence the result of cooperation between the hypnotist as well as his subject, not a form of power the hypnotist holds which can force the subject to follow his or her wishes.

After being under Hypnosis it is impossible to come out of the state on their own.

If you're in an hypnotist and they abruptly left the room two things can occur. You may either notice that the hypnotist has stopped speaking to you anymore and you will then awake feeling alert and fresh. It is also possible to fall to sleep, which is when you'll wake up in several moments (or many hours). The subject will get out of the trance all on his own.

Only those who are weak in their thinking are susceptible to being controlled.

False. Hypnosis does not have anything to do with willpower. Many people confuse hypnotibility with trustworthiness. There is no correlation between both. In fact, the more knowledgeable an individual is, the more easy it is to be attracted to. To be hypnotized, you need concentration imagination, vivid visualization and imagination.

In hypnosis, the person is completely unaware.

In all the time of a hypnotic process you'll be capable of hearing and think. You will be aware of the events happening within you. While your body may appear at ease, your mind is more alert than normal. A lot of people are concerned about stage hypnosis and also the reality that the participants frequently do bizarre actions during the session appear to be unaware of the world about the subject. The problem with this kind of activity is that it frequently scares away people who could actually benefit from hypnotherapy but fear losing control.

Under hypnosis, one could be convinced to divulge his secrets.

As stated above, when under the influence of hypnosis, the person is alert and actually more alert than in normal. The hypnotist is able to guide the subject to recall memories that have been lost. The decision of whether the subject will divulge these to the hypnotist is entirely at the discretion of the subject.

Hypnosis can be dangerous.

Untrue. The opposite is true. Hypnosis is a secure and natural procedure. One thing that people do not realize is that we experience Hypnosis many times throughout our everyday lives. For instance, when driving along the highway, most often people are shocked to discover that they've lost their consciousness for a few minutes. This is an instance of temporary hypnosis.

However, someone suffering from epilepsy should not be controlled by hypnosis.

You need special abilities to be to be hypnotized.

Anyone who has the will and the patience to learn can master the art of hypnosis.

As with other skills, like playing the piano or learning a new language, there are some who are "naturals" who are able to master their craft with minimal training While others may improve their skills through regular practice. A clear, confident voice is a plus but isn't a requirement. Of course, kids who lack an understanding and appreciation of the topic (usually younger than 5) might not react to hypnosis in a desired manner.

The user may be a dependent user of the hypnosis.

It is impossible to be dependent on the power of hypnosis since it doesn't have physical effect on the body.

But, many people are looking forward to the daily hypnosis sessions since they feel completely relaxed and feel refreshed.

A typical Hypnotic Session

A Hypnotic session is composed of three parts:

Induction:

Induction is the process of generating of a hypnotic trance within the person. As the body relaxes the body's metabolism as well as the brain's activity levels are decreased. This is the best condition to accept suggestions.

This is a crucial aspect of the process since when the body and mind do not are relaxed and relax, your conscious brain will keep filtering ideas into the subconscious because of the fact that it is analytical.

Programming:

This is the phase that the true benefits occur. As previously mentioned, the induction helps the mind prepare to program by removing the barrier between the subconscious and conscious mind.

The communicationthat is created lets the mind be fed positive thoughts by affirmations or images.

Awakening:

Once the subject has been given the desired programme the subject is taken into a trance typically, by counting between one and three or five.

Methods to induce Hypnosis

There are many methods of bringing hypnosis into one's subject, with the most well-known is body relaxation and creative relax (through visualization). Many hypnotists employ the combination of a variety of methods. An example of this is provided below. It is essential to keep in mind that no matter what method is employed the method must produce the following outcomes:

Relaxation of mind and body

The focus of attention is shifted to the left.

A lack of awareness of the external world and daily concerns.

A state of daydreaming that resembles trance.

The following script has been split into 2 parts: The Induction and Awakening. Follow the induction and then follow the instructions (given in the subsequent units). Then, you can take yourself out of the experience by through the Awakening. If you want to use it only for relaxation purposes then you can utilize it with no affirmations.

If you'd like you could request a person (with an excellent voice) to help you navigate any hypnosis exercise (using the scripts within this class) or even record it using your voice, and then practice the technique.

Induction:

"Close the eyes. then roll your eyeballs up and you can take 3 deep breathes and then let your body relax. Concentrate on relaxing every muscle in your body , from to the highest point of your skull all the way to those tips of your feet. Begin to relax. Begin to be aware of how comfortable your body is starting to feel. Your body is supported and you are able to let go and let your body relax. For a second, observe your calm, slow deep breathing. Take a deep breath and then exhale. Take a breath and then exhale. Every when you exhale, you feel more relaxed and comfortable.

For a deeper relaxation For a deeper relaxation, count backwards from twenty to one, you can visualize the number, if you wish.

Twenty . . . . Nineteen . . . Eighteen . . . Seventeen . .

Sixteen . . . . Fifteen . . . . Fourteen . . . Thirteen . . .

Twelve . . . . Eleven . . . . Ten . . . . . . Nine . . . . . Eight . . . . . Seven . . . . . Six . . . . . . Five . . . . .

Four . . . . . Three . . . . . Two . . . . . . One . . . . . "

[Insert programming if desired]

Awakening:

"Now I'm going to begin counting from 1 to 3 and at the point of 3 you'll be able to be able to open your eyes and feel fresh, light rejuvenated, vibrant delightful, happy and happy, and feeling much better than you did before. 1. Coming out slowly. 2. Yes, the album is out. 3. Open your eyes to feel fresh and rejuvenated, feeling joyful and cheerful and feeling better than you did before."

Guideline for proposing Suggestions and Programming:

Hypnotists utilize a variety of techniques to manipulate a subject's brain. Here is a list of these: (These techniques are to be integrated into the programming)

Affirmations:

In the state of relaxation that induces by hypnosis, the subconscious mind is very open to positive suggestions. These can be included in the program through carefully crafted affirmations. Studies show that when the body and mind are relaxed and relax, a reduction in brain's activity can open a direct access to the powerful subconscious mind, which allows for a faster and more effective methods of subconscious programming using thoughts that are not visible, and without interference from the conscious mind's analytical mind.

When forming AFFIRMATIONS, keep The following ideas in mind:

The affirmations must be clear as well as concise and clear.

They must be convincing and that the person is willing to accept.

They can be repeated for reinforcement.

Be positive. (For instance, use the phrase "You will remain punctual." Instead of using the word "you will be punctual."

"You won't be late.") Talk in the present in the present. ("You're improving your memory each day."

is significantly better than "You will notice the improvements within your brain.")

Visualization:

During the course, you might also imagine yourself reaching your objective.

Visualization is not the ideal method for either. It is better to daydream or wish. It's a sensible way to find and get everything you desire from your life. The practice of visualization helps you concentrate on what you desire, and assists in coordinating all of your available resourcesthat can be employed to help you achieve of your goal.

Trigger Words:

It is also possible to use trigger words to create a post the hypnotic conditioned reaction. In the hypnotic process it is possible to give your subconscious mind with specific phrases, which will serve as your conditioned response to create a specific behaviour. That is, anytime you want to act in a specific manner (for example, focusing on something you would like to read) All you need to do is shut your eyes and repeat the phrases to yourself.

Chapter 2: Re-Birth

The aim in this article is to explore another useful technique for hypnosis which is known as rebirth. The method is typically comprised of reliving the process of birth independently. The principal goal of this technique of the field of hypnosis is to make the subject aware of any emotions that are connected to the birth process and also to lift the person free of any trauma or difficulty he or she was aware of during the birthing process.

Evidence that Rebirth works

JM Schneck back in 2011, released the results of his research that showed that the technique of rebirthing is highly effective in getting the subject to relax and free of any trauma, if there is one. It's a highly efficient technique that can assist you in a variety of ways when used correctly.

A Short Story

One of my acquaintances has utilized this method for an individual suffering from anxiety and claustrophobia. In the course of applying the Re birthing techniques the patient was informed of that they had a traumatizing experience during their birth that they remember immediately that when they were born, they had their umbilical cords wrapped over their neck. The symptoms associated with the need for this method are eliminated once the effects of this procedure are relived physically.

What are the benefits of learning about re-birth?

It is important to understand what it takes to go through rebirthing, as it will assist you to relieve your patient of any trauma that's been present from the moment of their birth.

What do you need to Be Educated About Before Re-birth?

The main thing you need to be aware of regarding Rebirthing is that it's not essential that this procedure is limited to hypnotic therapy in a clinical setting. It can also be a part of physical process in nature. It can also assist in activating the birth feeling in the brain of your client.

How To do Re-birth

Step 1 : Write down an outline that will assist your subject to develop all the steps that were at play in causing his/her an emotional state during the time of their birth.

Step 2 : Make a checklist of the various methods that can aid you in getting using this technique.

Step 3 : Discover the most effective method of carrying out the technique in order to achieve positive results from it.

What Other Options Do You Have to apply Re-birth

The process of rebirthing could also be used on individuals who are analytical by nature and doesn't think of the opinions of others, however, they only focus on the things they're saying. This causes a mental trauma they suffer in their mind and is best treated with the method of Rebirthing.

Frequently asked questions and answers on Rebirth

Questions 1 and 2: How do I proceed happens if I used it for each age group?

Answer 1 : Yes , you could, but the only requirement that is required that the subject whom you're working must be able to fully comprehend what you are trying to get them to do. It will be more easy for you to enter inside the mind of your subject, and to respond according to their needs.

Question 2 : How do I employ this method professionally and what are the potential consequences of employing it in my work?

Answer 2: You can apply this method in your professional life , too however, you must first know the mindset of the topic you are working with.

Final Purport

The procedure and steps required to carry out the process of rebirth method have been explained clearly and further elaborated within this section. Also, you have learned various methods using this method.

Keys to Action Keys

Step 1 : Perform the process of rebirthing remembering the steps to begin with.

Action Key 2: Make sure that you're tackling this strategy in accordance with what your subject is thinking.

Chapter 3: What to Utilize Nlp to Overcome Social Phobia

The social phobia disorder is an disease that is felt by any person. Before tackling the ways to conquer the condition, it's best to understand what it means. Knowing the meaning of it will allow you to know if you or a loved ones or perhaps you suffers from social phobia.

Social phobia is described as a condition that is characterized by a constant and distinct fear of performance or social situations where humiliation could be a possibility. Being exposed to the act of the social situation almost invariably triggers an immediate anxiety reaction. Although adults and teenagers who suffer from this disorder have identified that their anxiety is unfounded it is not an issue for children. The majority of the time the social situations are averted, even though they are sometimes accompanied by anxiety. If you are less than 18 years old the symptoms should have been present for at least six months prior to the condition can be identified. However, this type of diagnosis should only be granted if the anxiety is accepted. It's like the context in which the stimuli , like being used in the class if the material is they are not prepared.

People suffering from social phobia can become hypersensitive in response to negative criticism negative feelings or words. They may also be unable to be assertive and suffer from lower self-esteem, or feelings of weakness. They could also be afflicted with weak social skills or indicators of anxiety. They also tend to are low on morale. However, this condition is not the only way to conquer it all. One way to overcome it is via Nuero Linguistic Programming. When you've learned about this strategy for the way to overcome social anxiety It is important to be aware of what it mean and how you can make use of it to overcome social anxiety.

NPL also known as Neuro Linguistic Programming is described as a 40 years old method that is believed to help people overcome negative beliefs and practices and enhances personal social life as well as business. However, there are some practitioners who make exaggerated claims about the efficacy. Many people have claimed they had overcome trauma experiences and fears through Neuro Linguistic Programming, frequent within a short amount of duration. Different strategies are used in order to achieve these results but they all depend heavily on the sensory experience and visualization.

What is the best way to utilize Nuero Linguistic Programming to overcome social anxiety? Here are some strategies to restore self-esteem

Representational Systems This is the method that allows for a variety of applications that increase motivation, emotional intensity , and relationship.

Mirroring and Matching: utilizing the characteristics of someone else's wording, structure, and other factors to form a the impression of a connection.

Moving Perceptual Spaces is similar to shifting from different viewpoints. It is a matter of three mental locations like self, the viewpoint of another person and an outsider's viewpoint.

Making Well-Formed Results Enhancing a particular sensory-based outcome. This includes a variety of possible applications, especially in the field of goal-setting.

State Management - This includes an array of systems that include changing physiological processes.

Reframing is to alter the context of an experience to alter its significance.

Meta Mode - this is an approach that incorporates many linguistic variations which aid in recognizing patterns of language which conceal the nature of the language through removal, modification, and generalization. This model can be effective in improving communication, and in helping to create the necessary changes.

The Swish Pattern is thought to be a highly effective method of replacing an unintentional, old behaviour with a more desirable desired behaviour. This type of method can be very effective in causing lasting changes in behavior and habits.

The above mentioned techniques are the fundamental or basic Neuro Linguistic Programming techniques that are employed to combat social anxiety. Because they are only the fundamental techniques that are available, there is an advanced technique that can be thought to be a successful one for conquering social anxiety. They are believed to be the most effective advanced methods for conquering social anxiety:

Meta-states are the mind-body state to accept another state to a higher-logical level, which is referred to as meta-states. It is certainly powerful to bring about a change in many areas for a particular person.

Nested Loops is the technique of linking states. It is a fantastic method to alter the state of other people while you interact with a particular individual or group of people.

Language Patterns are the linguistic tools that are used to enhance influence and improve communication.

New Behavior Generator is an idea-based method to know how to swiftly integrate new behaviors and skills.

They are the most powerful and advanced NLP which can be employed to conquer social anxiety. There are experts that can assist you with these methods. As a general rule of thumb that you should ask for help from those who are deemed to be competent to perform the job.

Chapter 4: Testing for Suggestions

Testing for suggestibility isn't an exam that is either pass or fail in the most fundamental sense. it is a sign of the level of trust you have with your subject. If a test is terribly wrong, then you're not matched with your subject. That is why after a few tests , you don't get the results you're looking for. Maybe the subject isn't making use of their imagination.

For these types of topics, research into an overload-style induction test should be conducted. In this article, we will go over the classic test of suggestibility. This is the lock hands.

There are three elements that will ensure the success of your suggestibility test:

1: Rapport.

2: Imagination.

3: Repetition.

This test can help increase compliance and improve the rapport. A successful test will reveal the level of rapport as well as trust, confidence, and completeness of your subject.

The most basic test:

"I want you to reach your arms out palms down. Now switch your hands so that they face each other, and bend your arms, press your palms together, and then interlock your fingers. I would like you to imagine there was a really strong glue in those palms, and as they press the glue gets closer and closer You are able to feel them sticking and locking more and more tightly joined. And now they're so tight that you can't take them apart even if you wanted to.

Now, I'm asking you to try pulling your hands apart. If you find that you aren't able to do it do it, now try and observe how much more you struggle and the harder they get. Do your best to break them up and then see if you can't."

Note the use of repetition and imagination however to increase the effectiveness of this technique, we make use of certain Advanced methods.

Utilizing time:

Begin by saying that your hands will be stuck. it is not noticed until you switch to hands that have been stuck. However, the change is noticeable.

Using dissociation:

Start by saying that your hands are stuck and you have not seen changing. Those hands are stuck, and the shift makes a significant difference.

The reason why this is all happening:

Three factors are needed to bring this working.

1. By placing your palms together, and then interlocking fingers, you create friction and pressure which makes it difficult to separate your fingers.

2. The imagery activates to stimulate the imagination, and when that imagination gets in the way of the power of imagination, it wins.

3. By building compliance and making sure that you prove is factual, they are willing to believe what you have said in the future.

This test of suggestibility can be used interchangeably with other tests.

Further Research: Google and YouTube: hypnotic phenomenon test for suggestibility arm lockout test pendulum test, test of suggestibility.

Chapter 5: Trance Induction Technique

Psychophysiological signs of trance include: mydriasis and gaze fixation slowing down blinking and swallowing reflexes decreasing the number of movements and muscle relaxation, slow and more rhythmic breathing, a decrease in heart rate and rate as well as smoothing facial muscles, and changing its color, attenuation of reaction to external sounds and ideomotor spontaneity, etc. One of the guidelines of Erickson trance is that if it's not, must behave like it's.

Guidance Trance Style that is based on the work of Erikson known as indirektivnym opportunity. Everyone feels the pressing necessity to protect their dignity and freedom. Therapists are just entering the world of human issues and is fully embracing its authenticity, and accepting it as it is. If the therapist believes that existing interpersonal relationships are established is established, he begins by draws attention to fragments of his own experience that are out of his mind, thereby giving him access to the resources are available, however, he is unable to notice.

According to Erikson To expand the human problem system and transform it into an answer to the system, you have to first be a part of a closed system issues and join in a way that you do not feel any differences between the patient and the therapy. It is an essential step to establish relationship. You can be tuned into any aspect of external human behavior. For instance, adjustment is feasible through "mirroring" or adjusting posture by synchronizing the rhythm of respiration speech, or joining the micromotion type of touch the chin while talking, etc.)

Consider, for instance, one of the methods of joining and preserving this formulation "X and X the formula X and X". Approval X is the approval for an agreement. This is an absolutely accurate assertion about the behavior changes that take place at the level of the client. Approval We: approval of reference, also known as an assertion that leads to a state of Trance. Example:

You are sitting on my couch (merger approbation).

And I am looking at you (joining applause).

You can breathe easily (merger approbation).

We're talking with you (connection acceptance).

Then you can begin to loosen (approval of authority).

Maykl Sparks, Ph.D. Professor, instructs students at the Faculty of Management Training at California State University in

Sacramento (California) disciplines that are related to human behavior within organizations. His management advice are offered to various organisations. The company also offers workshops in areas like training employees to work as a team and leadership, motivation, management, and communication. Particularly, he took part in the creation of a group training programs for the American astronauts that have been working in tandem in the orbital space station.

Specific techniques within the Ericsson theorizing

A number of specific strategies, a crucial link to the algorithm Erickson Hypnosis: dissociation between consciousness and insanity. Therapists must be able to construct complex sentences that exert some impact on the person by using the words "mind" as well as "unconscious" and as synonyms for those terms"in the background of consciousness" "in conscious awareness's background", "focus", "on the fringe of the attention."

Techniques employed in Erickson hypnosis trance to recycle and re-use, are universally applicable. They can be employed to induce trance and provide suggestions during the state of waking. There are six kinds in indirect speech messages: truisms, assumptions; questions and assertions to draw attention and to draw attention; opposition "A non-choice" and "the most appropriate decision". For instance, truisms can be used in situations where specific instructions from a physician are disguised as arguments. Assumptions (presubpozitsii) are a term is believed to clarify the existence of any thing or event and is used in phrases such as "The longer you are sitting on an armchair, the more you are entangled in the trance" or. There is no option: "You would like to go into a trance either with your eyes closed or shut." The result is that the client is free to select from a variety of possibilities, and each is very content with the therapy. When making the "right option" the therapist draws and the client's attention to the reactionthat prompts the person to dial"y," giving him full the freedom to choose. The patient is happy, and is beginning to comprehend that he shouldn't respond in a specific way.

One of the most popular methods used by Erickson for trance induction is hands that levitate. Simpler explanation of the process is like this. The patient relaxes and focuses on the emotions and sensations that are felt within your fingers. The therapist will demonstrate the option of not-legislative "imperceptible motions" in his hands and asks for a closer gaze at his hand trying to catch the moment that the movements become apparent. The suggestion is not of an authoritative kind of suggestion, but the client is interested to find out what will happen and will interpret the suggestion as a result of my personal experience, and relating his thoughts to the words of the psychotherapist. The first real suggestion - the client was told that one of his fingers moves first, with fingers separated and so on. This was followed by a further suggestions (one finger lifted and the rest of fingers follow by raising the hand and causing eye insomnia, fatigue suggestion etc.) If the hand of the client is raised, he stated that he would be asleep because the hand was elevated (mutual increasing). He suggested that he regulate the amount of time spent in the dream in order that when his hands touch to the skin, he was given the impression that he'd fell asleep because he had wanted to. In the end, the client slips into a state of trance.

A significant contribution to the evolution of self-hypnosis. Erickson believed in his technique was able to insert messages. The idea of Erickson was to create the suggestion in the form of text, and then to "dissolve" it into a sort tale content neutral, and then to indicate later some meaningful words that compose the message. In this scenario the therapist relies on the power to think associatively. Techniques that insert posts are the best way to induce consciousness. The concept of selecting, underlining messages is not unusual. As an idea, it's an essential element that human interaction. Methods of separating the messages inserted are different:

speech (change in the volume, speed, intonation of speech, the use of sound effects such as soputst Vyuschih-Speech and more.);

visual (gestures or gestures, changes in body posture, changes in face expressions);

Kinesthetic (touch the floor, the stroking, slapping, or similar);

Mixed (change in distance to that source point, mixing of the speech with that through-head alignment and the movement of sounds mixed, etc.).

The goal of dissociation of consciousness from unconsciousness is to is to learn how to construct complex sentences that will have an influence on the user. In this case it is a simple exercise on the structure of sentences. Utilizing the table, select an item from left hand side of the table. Then, attach the sentence any suggestions you have received from to the side on which you are. Then, after some time, begin to develop their own ideas.

1. Utilizing the table, Partner 1 makes a comment on the dissociation between consciousness and unconsciousness.

2. Partner 2 also makes use of tables, and provides a statement about the dissociation between consciousness and unconsciousness

3. Continue to switch. The exercise will last five minutes. Pay attention to the usage of words that are synonymous to "consciousness" as well as "unconscious": "in the front of consciousness""in the forefront of consciousness, "in in the background", "focus" - "on the outer edge of the attention."

Your mind's subconscious

1. Take note of what I'm saying. And

While

As

But 1. Do you have the ability to initiate making the necessary changes in your particular current state ...

2. It's possible that He would like to know what will happen in the coming days ... 2. Are you able to begin to recall the things that are the crucial to your life ...

3. You may be focussed on one or the other idea ... 3. Are you ready to begin

your journey that is unique and different to the norm.

4. Doubt the worth of what's happening right now. 4. I learned a lot and can apply the knowledge.

5. You can be aware of the is the kind of sensation you're currently experiencing. 5. It could have different ideas on what you'd like to achieve ...

6. Are eager to be right ... 6. Create images, you are kotoryepokazhutsya awe-in.

7. Are you aware of. What is taking place "here and today" ... 7. Increases understanding and understanding ..

8. It was a thought ... 8. Incorporated in more profound trans.

9. The attempt to comprehend the significance of what I'm saying ... 9. Attempts to understand the meaning of

what I'm talking about... Begin to grasp something crucial to you ...

10. kriticheskiotsenivaet and comprehend what is happening ... 10. The hidden wisdom is revealed. .

The use of stories and metaphors

Metaphor is a type of speech, which is the use of words and phrases in a symbolic sense, based on an analogy or similarity or comparisons. The concept of metaphor is based on the idea of similarity or similarity. it is a representation of the analogy in which X refers to Y, just as A belongs to B. To understand the significance of this metaphor, you has to increase the right hemisphere of their brain to ensure that the subconscious will be able to grasp the meaning that is desired.

The metaphor is identified by 4 "element":

the context or category,

an object that falls within a specific category,

the procedure of how this facility functions and

Applying this method in real-life situations or cross-checking the lines.

If we don't consider the philology for us, it's the metaphor can be described as an a fictional account of the client's circumstances. Figurative , so as to exclude literal analogies.

The most appealing aspect of this symbolism is the fact that it doesn't simply describes the situation however, it also suggests that there's the solution. It even provides the general direction. However, the information (the evidence and suggestion) provides the possibility of guessing as well as imagining and assuming that the client's motivation was precisely based on the experiences available to him and that he was and is pursuing.

The metaphor is profoundly symbolic. While we can discern symbols that are full of significance, but we don't or the client does not. Don't ask the client to ask questions. The client will determine its purpose. It's not always the case that we could should have thought of it before. The most important thing is that If the metaphor is constructed correctly, the user will discover the necessary (not always conscious) necessary meaning.

Tale-metafras you've readis characterized in the sense that every one we asked us after having read: "What is it?" Answered something unique and each time, Unrelated.

The metaphor for this should be:

A symbolic explanation of the overall nature of the issue.

A symbol of the principal actors (the characters)

Undefined symbol to resolve the issue.

The use of the symbol for vaguely described the nature of the proposed solution.

Reflection of the collision as the main incident.

Resolution: a strong emotional description of the way "everything will be okay" once the issue is settled for all the major forces operating.

General holiday.

What does this all means? We now know.

The core of the problem:

From the problem to its literal description, we follow three steps The formulation of the problem formulating the problem as a group as well as the formulation of problematic characters. For example that a man is Nedolyublen. And then to the world that is incredulous. The category of issues is the absence of value, vital to the quality of life. A symbol of being surrounded by a mountain range , a world of snow and cold, in which there is a lack of heat and sunlight.

characters:

In order to represent the characters you can imagine not only the metaphors of individuals however, you can also consider the emotions, forces abilities, qualities, and qualities. When you think of the inner "I" individual, we can look at these heroes- the personification of everything, and continue to go. It could become a mountain chain or a hero which blocks the passage of light and heat. It is possible to experience an idyllic fairy-tale summer with a sad face when she sees cooling her own home, where was once warm with her mighty bird that, in by overcoming obstacles, has made those living in cold regions know that right in the next corner, there is warmth ... and it goes on .

Decision:

It has to include "something". This isn't a concrete plan that is action-oriented, rather rather something that is ambiguous, yet also embodied by the hero or subject. The most important thing is whether it's a house is enchanted by fairies, a an unidentified bottle with an alcohol drink, a mysterious scroll or undiscovered road or another small wizard or the same bird, that can show the how ...

In addition, the re-read of "The Wizard of Oz" The Wizard of Oz: here as well as Goodwin, "great and terrible" Here and brains made from sawdust, silk heart and the determination to drink the characters, the symbols people ...

Application:

This is a delicate element that is part of the symbol. In reality, you are forwarding two or three vague sentences. The protagonist of "just" is given information on how to apply the symbol to his to make decisions. It is, however, the most important aspect of the idea that there's an answer, and it's possible to find a solution and it's a the most likely path. In our past, mountains, there is be talked about getting further than the mountains about the disenchantment of fairies, the long path to becoming a powerful wizard the necessity of sprinkle on a vial and a miraculous event occurred.

Event-conflict:

The typical client is heavy and hard. Also, it is important that you is expected to have a miraculous outcome. Yes, miracles do occur. However, it will happen within ... as soon when the hero will receive the bottle, will follow the route that convinces the wizard to travel through the mountains, or disrupt them.

If the purpose is not to embark for the difficult work of change, but rather to push for the obvious, and it's simple to make changes it is likely to be a contradiction: this is, as he puts it is a minor thing however, the consequences are.

There is another important aspect that separates metaphor from fairy tale and "adult" of love with "good" as well as "bad" male. We cannot be defeated. There must become "bad characters." In the first place, we don't know (though I've tried) which of the characters if they will tie to us as clients (and in addition, we do not identify with one or two, but can associate with a handful of). Furthermore, throughout the sequence of the story, I must discover that everyone - even the characters "bad" characters aren't so bad, but they all have their own issues and their own ideas of how to become "better." The more bizarre and unpredictably the story turns out to be, it is more surprising for all characters that will be more effective become the metaphor.

Thus, the destruction, humiliation, and defeat that the character in our story do not. It is a Miracle. After that, the hero takes the required (and frequently non-sensical) steps. For instance, not through fighting in the dark forest, he takes over the ravine and cleans it.

* "Do not shoot Prince Ivan. I'll still be of service!"

Resolution of the issue:

Take note of Carlson: "A miracle saved the life of one of my friends!" That's all it takes, this spirit should be the dominant metaphor. We describe vividly, with bright colors and in the joy, and then describe it - it was.

We do not discuss the enigma of the mechanism that is questioned. What is the best way to operate in general, we are simply forwarding. It is not our logic that is crucial, but - faith. The belief that miracles can happen might happen. There is hope. We accentuate the fact that work. Happened.

* "And that's how it went" ... "And when it was" ... "And in the exact time" ... "And as the final drop of water fell" ... Something took place. SOMETHING. It means ... it means that "all is good." Details and tears of joy to the faces of the characters. The narrator too.

Customers, may the joy of our customers be shared.

Celebration:

The next step is to complete the story, with faith in the most authoritative assertion about the reality that this didn't seem like a fairy tale to the heroes or all, as it was not in fact. This was the result that remained.

* "And they remained happily happy for the rest of their lives after."

The most common description is the holiday, during which there are many characters that are now close friends and have a reconciliation. Everyone has their own thing to do and they can make things right. Then, round and round the good things that began with Marvel.

It might find it interesting to create an analogy. But before you start make a note of the metaphor isn't necessarily a fairytale. This is a home story that concerns the neighbor or a client as well as "recollection" about "recently had a look at the story" and an adverb from the Gospel as well as the assumption of a sequence of "how it would be," and sometimes just three or two sentences for an example of comparison .

* "A friend of mine once put covered all the wool beneath shoulders in order to look acceptable, then picked it up at the

gym to strengthen your shoulders are aching.. Hoo, so you walk around the hall over two decades." It is a description of the method used in which customers make obsessed efforts to locate tangible evidence of their significance: the car, the office tie, car ... In this short article, it is all set. Take the steps apart if you wish.

Chapter 6: What to Do to Create Objective Goals that are realistic

Before you can achieve your goal, you have to have a plan to begin with. Most people don't have any goals in their lives and tend to drift along with the current. Because they lack focus in their lives, they don't accomplish much. If you have a friend who is someone like this you are likely to recognize that they are able to accomplish great things however they aren't focus-oriented and thus ineffective. However there are people who set their targets to such a level that it is difficult to reach them. This kind of person becomes depressed and tense for the duration, because they constantly fail.

Any goal that hasn't been accomplished is a loss. If you do succeed in achieving the goal you set and you are disappointed that it took more time than it really did. If you're that kind of person, then chances are you're not able unwind, and you push yourself all the time. In this scenario you can accomplish quite a bit but you won't take pleasure in the process. Failure to accomplish your goals when you had hoped can hinder you from enjoying the accomplishments. The aging process begins before you reach your age and your vitality and energy gets sucked up by anxiety and stress. Depression is the result of your disillusionment and despair and.

In both of these cases there is a problem that's common to all, and that's the inability to set realistic goals that will help you navigate your way through life. If you're the type who moves with the flow and has a tendency to have very little or zero goals. This is usually due to the fear of failing. You've learned that failing causes anxiety and depression and, if you don't set a objective, you are not able to fail. Unfortunately, both scenarios end up in defeat.

Alongside setting high or low targets, you may be setting targets that's so complex that you don't know whether or not you've achieved your objectives. If this happens, because you're not able to establish your goals and you aren't able to determine when you've accomplished them, you immediately think that you failed. You could, for instance, determine that the goal you have set in life is becoming successful, and therefore spend all of your energy and time in pursuing success. If you are asked to define what you consider success all you have to offer is some vague notion however you know that if you observe it, you'll be able to know it.

The reality is, there's no any such thing as success. What you can get is a few small successes, as opposed to some mythical notion known as success. If you haven't accomplished this it is your responsibility to set realistic and good targets for yourself. They will give guidance for your life and give you a sense of accomplishment and satisfaction as you reach them.

There are two kinds of goals: long-term and short-term goals. These are the most important goals you wish to accomplish in your life at the end, while short-term objectives are what you have to achieve at least at the moment. To achieve your long-term goals, you must accomplish a number of small-scale goals that lead into the larger one, for instance enrollment in college, selecting the appropriate classes, passing your tests in a reasonable amount of credits and obtaining a college degree and then gaining employment.

Here are some tips to help you establish excellent long-term goals

Determine if the goal is suitable for you. Beware of goals that are not clear enough or too high or are too low. It may be beneficial to speak to others and learn from their experience. Find friends or experts and ask for advice on what is the most realistic objective for you.

Generalize your long-term objectives, instead of setting them in a specific way. Setting them as specific means you're making yourself vulnerable to failing. However when you set them as general goals they can be achieved in many different ways. For instance, it's more sensible to strive to contribute to the well-being of your community rather than try to be as the most exceptional citizen.

Once you've decided on your long-term goals, you should analyze it in relation to the short-term goals you need to reach to reach it. Find out the direction your short-term goals must follow. In the majority of cases there's usually more than one method to achieve a long-term goal. There is no requirement to follow the route that somebody else has taken. You are free to pursue it in the way that you think is most comfortable for you.

*Start now. Get started on immediate goals. Establish a realistic schedule and keep in mind that goals worth doing usually take time. Many people underestimate the time required to reach the desired goal. It is crucial to be patient otherwise you'll feel nervous, stressed and angry.

Here are some guidelines to help you establish good short-term goals.

Short-term goals must be achievable, similar to the long-term objectives. It is important to make them tiny and distinct, in order that they lead toward the ultimate goal. You must be able to achieve these tasks more or less in a matter of minutes.

They must be more specific. It is important to define them enough that you will be able to identify your next steps, and also the direction you're taking.

You should organize and plan your plan for reaching these goals for the short term so that you're more likely to accomplish them.

In the event that you fail to meet one of your goals for the short term, be careful not to magnify it out to the point of being out of context. If you've been unsuccessful or have made a mistake does not mean you'll never be able to achieve your final objective. If you fall short of the short-term goals, take a step back and try another time, or find an alternative way around the problem.

Celebrate every time you accomplish an immediate target.

Psychologists define this as rewarding your self to do something you want to and it's extremely efficient. It isn't necessary to be rewarded with something extravagant.

Let's suppose, for instance you're doing your homework for an exam. It is possible to place some nuts or candy on the table and break up the content you're reading into smaller sections, such as the basics or sections of a chapter or pages. You can reward yourself with a piece of nuts or a piece of candy each when you finish the section. It is best to keep the units as small as possible and to set regular rewards.

It's not always efficient to give massive rewards following a long period of effort. It is possible to apply this principle to any job. But, this doesn't necessarily mean that you should not give yourself a reward after having completed an important job. If you have completed an entire semester or course reward yourself to a quick getaway, a costly dinner, or a type of reward. If you organize your life in this manner you'll enjoy your life regardless of what you're doing.

Once you've established your short and long time goals, you can set them up in your subconscious mind by following the guidelines for implementing autosuggestions. After this is done you should not be focusing on your goals.

If you place too much emphasis at your goal, you'll discover that you are too focused on the future to be present in the moment - constantly traveling without a goal. Thinking too much about the future may cause you to be unhappy in the present and eventually commit unwise sacrifices to reach your goals. If you're always focused on your goals for the future and planning to look forward to the next decade, then the time may never arrive.

Planning and direction when you set goals. After you've set the goals, you must keep them in an end of your head and pay more attention to the current.

The process of entering Hypnosis

Close your eyes and try to get rid of any anxiety or worry out of your thoughts. It may be impossible to not think once you begin. Thoughts may continue overtaking your mind however, when you do, don't force thoughts to go away. Recognize them as unbiased and then allow them to go. A few people choose a spot on the wall and then pay attention to the area. It could be a spot of smudges or the corner or whatever you want the point to appear. Focus on the issue by focusing your eyes. Repeat to yourself that they're getting more and more heavy, and let them close when you're not in a position to open them for long enough.

Recognize the tension within your body. Starting with your toes and think of the tension disappearing slowly away from your body, and disappearing. Imagine it dissolving from each of your body's parts by one at a time starting with your toes and then spreading upwards through your body. Imagine all the body parts of your body getting lighter and less heavy as you become liberated from tension.

Relax your feet and toes and move on to your calves, hips stomach, thighs and so on. until all parts in your body have been at ease, including your head and face. It is also possible to use visualization techniques that focus on something you love or find relaxing or soothing, such as water, to increase the enjoyment. Enjoy the sensation of water flowing across your feet and ankles and washing away tension.

Take slow, deep breaths. When you breathe out, visualize the tension and negative energy dissipating through a cloud of darkness. Inhale, and imagine the air returning as a vibrant force brimming with vitality and energy. When you reach this point it is yours to visualize however you want. Imagine an apple and cut it in quarters within your mind. Imagine the pieces breaking apart, and then falling on the plate. Place it in your mouth... What's your reaction? What does it smell as well as taste and feel? Now, you can move to visuals that have more meaning. Imagine yourself running off those weights. Imagine your debts blowing away in the breeze. Input as much detail that you are able to. Keep all five senses on your your mind.

Accept the fact that you're now totally at ease. Imagine yourself standing at an eminent point on a set of ten steps that is beginning to sink into the water on the 5th step. Imagine every aspect of the scene in your head from the top to the bottom. You can imagine that you'll be to the bottom of the stairway beginning at 10. Keep each number in your head. Imagine yourself getting closer to the bottom of the stairwell every time you count down. Imagine the sensation of every step you take as you count them down below your feet. When you get at the 5th step try to imagine and feel the cold water and imagine yourself entering an oasis of cleanness and pureness. When you begin to descend the remaining five steps, you will feel the water rising upwards throughout your body. You should feel a little numb and you may notice a faster heart rate. But just accept it and let any concerns about the situation to go away as the water.

Experience a floating feeling. When you get to your lowest point in the lake it is unlikely that you will be feeling anything, other than feeling like you are floating in the air. You may even feel as though you're spinning. If you don't feel this, attempt again however, at a slower pace while trying to comprehend what's happening. If you can attain this state it is possible to solve your issues and decide what you would like to achieve from the point you're at.

Start narrating what you're doing right now, and speak to yourself in both the present and future in a way that you're reading from the page. Imagine that there are three boxes in the water , which you must swim through to get to. The boxes should be opened slowly after you've located them in one step at a. When you open each box begin to tell yourself the events that are taking place. For example, "As I open this box, I see a bright light coming over me, it is becoming element of myself. This is my newfound confidence that's now integral part of my being, which means I'll never forget it."

As a guideline, avoid making statements that have an negative significance, such as "I do not want to be tired and angry." Instead you could use the phrase, "I am becoming cool and relaxed."

Repeat your affirmations positive repeatedly as often as you'd like. You could also begin to wander through the water as you empty the boxes and uncover treasures that can be found in self-confidence, money and other things, or simply relaxing your tensions. Find the areas in which the water is hot and cold or brimming with wildfire and then allow your imagination to run wild.

Make preparations to break out of the state of hypnosis. Continue climbing the steps and then out into the ocean until you've completed the fourth step again. When you're removed from the water and on to the 6th step you might feel heavy or feel like you're carrying something on your chest that is weighing you down. Keep your eyes on the step until you feel lighter, and continue you repeat your affirmations of positive energy continuously.

Continue up the stairs until it is completed, visualizing the steps in order of their numbers, and imagining the steps beneath you. Once you reach the top, allow yourself some time before waking up. Imagine yourself opening a doorway to the world. Slowly imagine the light coming in from the opening. The eyes should now be open naturally. You may also count to 10 if you have to, and tell yourself your eyes should be opened automatically after you have finished. Make sure to take your time getting up and then repeat to yourself what you usually tell yourself when you get up such as, "wide awake!" This will help bring your brain to its conscious stateand bring you return to the reality.

Improve Your Experience with Hypnosis

This means that it is impossible to create any self-hypnosis when you're not open about it. In order for it to work it is essential to be confident in yourself as well as the actions you take. If you're serious about your intentions you will succeed. If you're not successful the first attempt don't erase it immediately. Re-visit it in several days, and re-visit the lessons. Some things require some time to adjust to and perfect.

Be open-minded You must believe in the possibility of this happening for it to be successful. Your progress is slowed by any doubts you might be facing.

Try to test yourself physically. If you want to prove you're in a state of trance, there are exercises you can do to demonstrate this. Anything that you feel or can see could be effective. Here are some tips to explore:

Intertwine your fingers and hold them together throughout your trance. Try convincing yourself that they're locked together. Then try to break them. If you discover that you're not able to... you have evidence!

Imagine one of your arms becoming heavier and heavier. It's not necessary to select one; your brain will automatically take over the task. Imagine a book with it at the top. Now, attempt to lift it. Does it seem feasible?

Visualize the situation The issue is not what you're trying to achieve - whether that is positive thinking or losing weight, confidence or anything else... Just imagine yourself in the scenario and react as you were there to reactor behave the way you'd like to be. If you're trying to shed some weight, imagine yourself in those slim jeans in no time, looking at your gorgeous body when you look in the mirror.

Most people utilize self-hypnosis to conquer certain challenges such as shyness. There's no need to confront the issue directly and do anything else that you can work. Simply picturing yourself running your job with your head held high looking at your partner and smiling could be the first step toward an energised and confident you.

Utilize other things to assist your experience: Many people prefer using music to help to hypnotize themselves. If a specific scene like the forests, water, etc., would help the process, it is readily accessible. Timers can be useful also. For some people, it is difficult to come out of a Trance and eventually getting lost in the flow of the time. If you don't want get hypnotized for a long time it is possible to take advantage of an alarm clock. Be sure to select an uplifting tone that will get you from the trance.

Utilize this exercise to enhance yourself: Pick an objective you'd like to achieve, concentrate on it during your relaxation. Consider who you want to be and become the person you want to be. Hypnosis is a great tool for deep, meditative meditation, but it's superior in the sense that you can utilize it to achieve a larger and more beneficial reason.

Once you're mentally and physically ready to enter the state of hypnosis the following step will be to get yourself in a Trance. But before we get into the details about that, let's discuss some of the most important mental rules you must be aware of when you get ready to enter the trance.

Chapter 7: Altered States

Many people associate the concept of "altered states" with mind-altering substances. Although the two terms are frequently employed in conjunction however, they could and frequently refer to distinct events. Drugs are among the numerous ways that one can attain an altered condition. Since many people abuse substances, this may not be a beneficial or healthy method of to enter into a state of altered.

If someone is looking to improve their life, there are many different ways to achieve our state of being. Let's examine some examples...

HYPNOSIS

Most people, regardless of whether you choose to use self-hypnosis or consult a hypnotist the first goal is to attain an altered level of enhanced possibility. The mind is able to let go of its inhibitions and allows you to more easily believe in the positive thoughts you receive. This allows the hypnotist , or for self-hypnosis, your own script you've written, to basically direct your unconscious mind.

Because this is a book about hypnosis we'll stop here for the moment, and then explore other ways of altering your mind.

Meditation

The practice of meditation is typically connected to monks, mystics, and other spiritual practices, but you don't need necessarily be monk, mystic or monk to reap the benefits of meditation. It's true that you don't need to live in a specific area to practice it. You can practice it in your living room or even while walking.

The goal for meditation is rid your thoughts of continual bombardment of negative distractions that we all encounter. It's the loud neighbors, chatty officemates, city traffic , and spam that isn't needed. It allows you to calm your mind so that the distractions are able to gently drift off. You'll feel relaxed and at ease.

The expression "meditation" is a reference to a state of mind where your mind and body are at peace and conscious. One of the most effective ways to contemplate meditation is to consider it as an exercise in discipline. Many people believe that meditation is an attempt to clear your mind it's not the only possible goal. My personal practice is mindfulness meditation. The purpose for mindfulness meditation is be constantly mindless. When thoughts are passing through your mind, you make note of them. This can help you discover and deal with unwelcome thoughts and ideas.

Whatever kind of meditation you do It has been demonstrated to be extremely beneficial in developing mental discipline. It accomplishes this by giving you the mental tools that you can employ to remain at peace, regardless of what sort of situation you're in.

Lucid Dreaming

Lucid dreaming is a form of dreaming that you as the dreamer are aware of the fact that you in a dream. It allows you to direct the direction of your dreams. You can use your dream as a test ground for experiences you wouldn't have otherwise experience to help you heal or for other reasons.

HYPNAGOGIA

Although lucid dreams can be beneficial, not all people are capable of lucidity during their dreams. In addition it requires some time and practice. For the majority of people, it's simpler to maintain the state of "hypnagogia," which is the time before you go to sleep. When you are in this state, it feels to like you're not asleep but still not awake.

Many of the greatest thinkers, such as such as Thomas Edison, are said to have used this method to come up with ideas as it places a person in a state that is heightened imagination. The good part about hypnagogia, is that it's a great kind of altered consciousness that can be utilized to improve your self-development. Most likely, you're experiencing this state at least every day!

Martial Arts and Physical Sports

Many people are able to enter into an altered state through the practice of martial arts or other sports like rock climbing sky diving or surfing, skateboarding, and many other sports that require the highest levels of physical skill and mental focus. Many of them will strive to get so proficient in these sports that their minds enter "the zone" where they are in a zone of super-heightened but calm awareness. The result is that being in the zone lets them achieve incredible physical feats.

They are just as mind-altering as other drugs. These activities trigger the brain to naturally create substances that are similar to the drugs people take to get the sensation of a "high."

Chapter 8: Ideas Suggestions...

In a state of hypnosis, your body is at a low level and your mind is open to suggestions. These suggestions are sent directly to your subconscious mind and affect your actions without effort. If you're able to make use of hypnosis successfully, targets like stopping smoking, work out more and rest better, and feel more comfortable in social situations can be achieved with little effort.

I'm sure you've successfully gotten yourself into a relaxed state of trance effortlessly. You might be able to get both in and out of neutral hypnosis without the aid of a timer. Therefore, you must be prepared to begin giving yourself suggestions. There are three methods you can achieve this, and I'll explain them in greater detail. You might already know what objectives you'd like to accomplish through hypnosis. However, keep in mind that no matter how wonderful an instrument as it might be, it won't do the job over night. It would be fantastic for you to go into an hypnotic state and be told that all your worries will disappear when you awake from an euphoria. Sorry to disappoint you, but that is not the way hypnosis works. It is essential to understand what you are working toward, develop an action strategy using the power of hypnosis. When you're ready take action, you must read the following article.

The Anatomy of an Idea

Hypnotic scripts come in various lengths, depending on the requirements of your. It could be a single sentence, or a couple of short sentences or even a whole narrative. No matter how long the script is it is, all hypnotic scripts have the same general format. This is the contents of an idea, but in no specific order:

The ultimate goal

The solution is a sequence of steps

A specific command

Before you formulate any type of suggestion, make it sure you know what you'd like to accomplish and the way you'll be getting there. Record that in your hypnosis journal. Always begin with the end in mind , and then be specific. For instance, if the intention is to shed weight, make it clear what weight you would like to shed.

The examples below are intended to provide guidance and you aren't required to adhere to the exact wordings. You are welcome to alter them to fit your specific situation and requirements.

Short and Concise Tips

I'm going to get the process by creating a two or one-sentence suggestion. This kind of suggestion is the most efficient when you need to incorporate a simple behaviour into your routine to help you achieve your goals. It's as close as an easy fix that you can get by using the power of hypnosis.

To demonstrate the concept, I will make use of two distinct instances to illustrate. Let's start with the first instance: the aim of getting more active. You're aware that simply going for a walk in the local park for about an hour, preferably every week, a couple of times could be a great way to reduce your lifestyle of sedentary. Here's how to come up with a plan and then implement it:

1. Set a goal for yourself (Walk for an hour each day for a total of four days).

2.Think of a new way that will help you achieve your desired goal. It could be something you are able to do differently from your schedule (Spend less time at your computer).

3.What are two ways you can take to help you to stick with the new plan of behavior? (Cut the time you spend on internet surfing, and then take an afternoon stroll in the nearby park.)

4.Write an essay that directs you to complete the two tasks in step 3. (I will switch on my computer for about an hour, and then make use of that time to go for some time in the parks.)

5.Add the purpose into your statement. (I will go for a walk four times each week, and turn off my computer for one hour before heading towards the parks.)

6.Add a specific instruction to your sentence. It's a sort of an affirmative act. (I will walk every day for four days of the week, and turn off my computer for an hour before heading towards the parks. So, I'll go to the park in the evening of every Monday on Wednesday, Friday, and Sunday. I will not even go on social media while walking).

7.Once you have your idea developed, induce hypnosis. Then repeat the sentence as you're in a state of hypnosis. You are free to repeat the idea for as many times as you'd like. Once you have said it, picture yourself doing the things you mentioned. Spend time to visualize yourself reaching your goal. Sessions could be as long, or shorter as appropriate.

8. Then, you can add an affirmative affirmation along with an awakening thought. Make it clear after you have clearly visualized having accomplished your objective of gently bringing yourself out of the hypnosis. (Now having taken in the ideas I will pay attention to my mind and body with five, and then open my eyes.)

It is possible to apply the suggestion the duration you require. Remember to keep it in your hypnosis journal. When you feel that you've achieved your goal and are willing to move onto another, you may want to go again from the beginning or set a target that builds on your previous one. Let's take a look at another scenario following the same process that we have already discussed and this time, for the problem of falling asleep:

1. The ultimate goal is to sleep easily.

2.Decide on a new habit such as mindfulness meditation. It can be practiced for 15 minutes every day.

3.Two things that can simplify the process You can listen to soothing instrumental music prior to bed and then learn to concentrate on your breathe for 15 mins.

4.Give yourself some guidelines If I am going to bed each evening, I will listen to relaxing music and concentrate only on my breathing for fifteen minutes.

5.Add your goals You can say: I'll sleep quickly if I take the time to enjoy some peaceful music, and then focus in my breathing during fifteen minutes prior to bed each night.

6.Add an explicit command for example: I'll fall asleep quickly if I take the time to listen to calm music and focus in my breathing during fifteen minutes prior to bed each night. I will relax and meditate to make it easy for me to fall asleep afterwards.

7.Induce the state of hypnosis by saying suggestions, and visualize the picture of successful outcomes.

8. Stop the script and session by offering a wake-up suggestion.

The Solution is in the script

If you're dealing with a problem that is more complicated with multiple layers of solution are required, use an extended script that has an entire narrative. The process of entering the hypnosis process and implanting suggestions is similar however the script takes longer time to process and visualize. This method is most effective for emotional problems in which you are not in control over the circumstances, other than how you respond to it in the most effective way that you can. In this instance I will make use of performance anxiety as the main issue.

If you don't earn a living from public speaking or on a the stage, it's not surprising that nerves can get the over you. The technique I'm about explain to you is widely employed in sports, where athletes are usually trained to visualize the best outcomes in their work. This technique can be applied in any similar situation regardless of whether you need to master an interview or stop the emotions of your mind from getting over you prior to an unpleasant encounter. My only suggestion is to plan prior to the event, or at least allow yourself a minimum of 24 hours prior to the event you are planning to attend to practice self-hypnosis.

The hypnotic script that you create should include the following aspects:

1. The issue

2.The solution

3.Steps to reach the answer. The goal is to limit the number of steps to three at most.

4.Visualizing the steps in one step at a and in great detail using all the senses

5.Visualizing the scenes of success

6.Coming out of the hypnosis

Begin by taking the time to think about your thoughts and record precisely what you are struggling with. Make your issue clear. For example the problem statement reads, "I am worried that my presentation about the latest product of the company at the convention in coming weeks isn't engaging and thorough sufficient." Solution might be "I should be prepared to ensure that my audience is fully engaged."

Here is a script sample for making a presentation

The steps to solving the problem:

1. I will review my plan to present with the team leader so that I've covered all the important points.

2. I will practice my presentation with the group to increase my confidence.

3. I will be asking for their honest feedback as well as areas where I could improve.

Then, induce hypnosis. imagine yourself completing the steps that lead to your solution. Make sure you don't just look at the scene as if it were a movie in your mind's eye, but also to feel the smell, hear, as well as taste the scene. Next, you can visualize the scene of your success in all its details.

Based on the example above imagine yourself walking onto the stage and show the audience your face. You're calm as well-prepared, and you are ready to take on the stage! You can feel the cool breeze in the hall of the convention and sip a glass of water prior to speaking . You can see yourself giving your presentation, navigating each slide onto the overhead screen. The audience will respond with laughter to the occasional jokes you have made while the way. Talk about your product. After the presentation, thank your audience, and they applaud. When you leave on stage, your audience is there to thank on a job completed. When you think about the whole thing, you can you feel the joy that is rising in your. End your meditation by saying your wake-up call to lift you out of the stupor.

Do hypnosis guarantees success? No but it does improve your chances and make you more mentally prepared. There is nothing worse than being under pressure and experiencing a anxiety crisis before even beginning. When you use hypnosis, your goal is to develop a mental roadmap to achieve success. If your mental blueprint is one of 'I'm not capable do it', what's the probability of the actual situation manifesting as 'I am able to I can'? By using hypnosis to boost faith in your self, you will find that the fight is already half-won.

Make an Story

Have you ever watched a film or read something that makes you want to know more about the plot? Did you ever feel compelled by the story? Have you ever had a story caused you to question what you already knew? It's hard to identify the source but there's something in the story that makes you smile. Stories are a favorite of ours and stories more than hard facts and figures for a reason . A well-told story is a type that suggests something indirect. The unconscious mind is great in deciphering things in a symbolic way when the analytical and critical conscious mind doesn't get involved.

This method of making suggestions is an extremely advanced one, and requires more time and effort for implementation. This also requires you to push your imagination to think of an idea, which is the most intriguing kind of suggestion. Instead of offering ideas with instructions and directives then you'll be telling yourself a story that is metaphorical while under hypnosis. This is followed by visualisation. The best use of metaphoric stories is to develop a different mindset, perception or belief. For example, if you are not confident and feel awkward in social settings Perhaps you think that because of who that you are, you'll never be able to attain acceptance and love or create a mindset that will lead to bettering your financial situation These are the types of situations in which a metaphoric story, when repeated under hypnosis would be the best.

A metaphoric tale is more effective when it's given to you by someone with a clear comprehension of your situation and can create an intriguing story full of symbols. So, you can let the indirect ideas take in without pondering the implications. In the next chapter, you'll learn how to hypnotize others, and the ability to craft the illusion of a story comes in useful. If you're interested in giving this method of making suggestions try, there's absolutely no harm in testing it yourself.

There is no set of guidelines to come up with a story that is metaphorical You can simply play around with it! Begin by thinking about stories that inspire you, particularly folklores and fairy tales, perhaps revisiting the books or films that you like. Disney stories contain a lot of symbolism and characters that you could take on.

I will give an easy example of developing self-confidence and self-motivation. Imagine that you face a daunting task in front of you that could only describe as an "uphill struggle". It's certainly not a difficult feat to accomplish however, it definitely presents an obstacle that you're not certain of being in a position to conquer. It is possible to make use of a mountain's slope as a metaphor for your story. When you are hypnotized imagine yourself at the bottom of a mountain, preparing to race to the summit. Along the way the three obstructions are that look like an obstruction in the form of a boulder and a river that you must traverse, and a unstable bridge - each symbolizing something that is hindering you. The boulder may represent limitations in views, the river could represent social expectations, and the bridge could be an anxiety about failure.

You can also add affirmative ideas for example, "I will clear whatever obstacles I face. I am certain of success." Next, imagine yourself running along the mountain's slope and stopping at every obstruction, where you'll find ways to get over the obstacles. After you have conquered each obstacle you will arrive at the magnificent palace at the top of the mountain which is where a person waits to meet you. Since this is your personal story, that person could be anyone you've met, the metaphorical persona for your feelings and a fictional character or perhaps your future self! What would they say to you? What kind of reward will they offer you in return to thank you for your work? It's your choice to choose.

For the end of your session you may reaffirm the goal to conclude your session, and then follow it up with your awakening suggestion. You could phrase it like, "I have removed all obstacles that hinder my success. If I reach the number five I'll turn my attention back to my body and mind."

Create yourself your own tapes for hypnosis

Once you've learned how to make suggestions, I'm going to guide you through a second method to make your self-hypnosis experience more enjoyable. The most effective way to offer yourself suggestions while hypnotized is to remember the script you've created for yourself prior to entering the state of hypnosis, and then repeat it to yourself once you're under. This is most effectively when suggestions are small but it can be quite difficult when you are working using a long script. If that's the situation, you can record your voice while reciting the script and then play it back to yourself. With the voice recording function on the majority of cellphones, you can record audio and then have it transferred onto your computer or MP3 player.

Making your own hypnosis recordings is a bit of planning. in case you're not accustomed to using the recording device it may require some time and practice. I would highly suggest you create a carefully written script. The majority of hypnotic audio tracks on the market run a time of between 30 minutes and an hour, and they guide the listener from beginning to end. Therefore, if you intend to create your own hypnosis tapes prepare a complete plan for your entire process which includes suggestion, induction and visualization guides and reawakening. Then, record the entire session. Utilize a soft, low tones of voice.

Be patient and keep practicing

I sincerely hope that you're able to utilize the power of hypnosis in ways that help you accomplish what you've never imagined possible. If you've achieved significant improvements in trying to resolve a long-standing issue as you learn self-hypnosis techniques, give yourself an earful since you're definitely on the right track! If you're feeling like you're not progressing do not give up! Hypnosis isn't a one-touch solution. It will take time to master your mind however, it will be worth it.

Chapter 9: Limits of Self Hypnosis

Self-hypnosis is best employed as a tool, not as a method to get away from reality. A lot of things is, as the old saying goes, is harmful. Self-hypnosis may cease being beneficial and is destructive.

The main drawback to self-hypnosis is its fact that the entire the techniques involved in achieving the hypnotic state are carried out in the exact same way by the same individual. To master the art of self-hypnosis requires a significant amount of practice and time are necessary to master the skill and be able to execute consistently. The process of entering an hypnotic state that is self-initiated is quite simple, however it is a bit of effort necessary when you need to utilize this method for reaching your objective. Many people try repeatedly and when they fail to see any change , they abandon the effort. This is a mistake and an insufficiency when it comes to self-hypnosis. The people who learn to use self-hypnosis must be patient and persistent since the effects of self-hypnosis are cumulative and require repeated sessions to see the results.

A large number of people try self-hypnosis and, after not seeing any major change or effect will decide to stop self-hypnosis. Some of the explanations given for the low success rate of self-hypnosis are:

Someone might not have the knowledge to fully comprehend the nature of their problem

The research has demonstrated that the capability to assist yourself will only be as effective as your ability to remain open and honest about is the nature of the issues that need to be resolved. The process of identifying these issues can be difficult if you don't know the nature of these issues. A clear and accurate evaluation or judgement is needed on the problems that need to be tackled, however the majority of people lack the perception and objectiveness. There are many reasons and methods of denial or denying the reality of the situation, even in situations where such denial doesn't help their long-term goals in their lives. You may be denial about your troubles and your defense mechanisms or strategies for denial make it difficult for you to discern the causes and the root cause. Since you can't solve what you don't know and you won't be able to resolve your issues through self-hypnosis. It is possible that you will create new problems rather than solving them.

Someone may not have the expertise to solve your issues

A different challenge that anyone could face is working out the best way to resolve the issues that they face. This is particularly the case for those who are honest and precise in their understanding of the root of their difficulties. In order to be successful in self-hypnosis, the person needs to possess accurate information. The information is about what causes problems and how to fix the issues that are identified. be addressed. The issue is that you need access to resources as well as the desire to study and read the sources before you are able to solve the issue. The majority of people aren't born with the expertise on how to solve problems, and not everyone is prepared or ready to do the effort.

A person may not have the motivation to continue using self-hypnosis

This is another issue that a person faces when doing self-hypnosis. A lot of people know what they are expected to do in self-hypnosis, but fail to adhere to the program. Making and maintaining the desire to stick to self-hypnosis is one of the biggest issues.

Other limitations of self-hypnosis include:

Being obsessed or failing to make the most of self-hypnosis: Individuals are likely to fall into the routine of attending a hypnosis session every day to the point where the brain doesn't get the chance to re-connect and absorb the knowledge gained in the hypnotic state. Self-hypnosis shouldn't be practiced more than five days one week.

Self-hypnosis might not be at a place to resolve many of the issues that a person may be facing. Problems that are complex and can affect an individual at an extensive level and can cause immense personal distress must be dealt with by a professional. Issues like depression or trauma as well as destructive behaviors will require that individuals seek professional assistance that combines counseling with individualized therapy.

There is debate over what is more effective professionally-managed hypnosis and self-hypnosis. The efficacy of any form of hypnosis is different depending on how individuals respond to sessions. One critique that self-hypnosis may receives is that it doesn't always lead to change in behavior.

Self-hypnosis doesn't affect the body's structure in ways that go beyond the scope of. Therefore, it is not an accurate assumption that self-hypnosis will aid in gaining inches in size, get rid of cancer or shed excess weight. Self-hypnosis can be used to facilitate changes put into the body by the person who is hypnotized however these changes are restricted to physical processes. For instance, self hypnosis is not a cure for cancer, but it can aid in reducing the negative effects of treatments like chemotherapy. Hypnosis can definitely aid in feeling more relaxed and balanced physically.

Chapter 10: Neuro Linguistic Programming (Nlp)

NLP A brief overview

1970 saw the emergence that led to the development of Neuro Linguistic Programming (NLP) by John Grinder and Richard Bandler.

The three major human experiences are described in the title itself. The neurological processes we perform, as well as our capacity to communicate with written and spoken language, and programming learning, education, and social structures and systems of social organization are what distinguish us from other animals. Our bodies have extremely complex neurologic pathways that control the way our bodies function. As humans we can communicate in a complex way with other people. The models we develop from education, engineering to community, are the hallmarks and maybe an in-depth analysis of the two other facets of of this school of study. NLP is an attempt to understand and deconstruct the interactions in the brain as well as the languages we employ. Through this understanding it is possible to recreate those processes to better assist individuals.

What exactly does NLP try to accomplish? It's a fact that we do not utilize our brains to the fullest capabilities. It's that the majority of us are only using about 10% of our brain's capacity. NLP can assist you in increasing your brain's overall performance and, consequently, your efficiency in your daily life, particularly at work. Through the use of NLP you are able to attempt to achieve excellence in specific areas or gain the whole-person growth. However, NLP is also used by hypnotherapists for treating a variety of ailments that are physical and psychological. Fundamentally, NLP posits that through the process that comes from "modelling" (taking into account the characteristics of models) it is possible to be ourselves exceptional.

NLP relies on a certain amount of individual intelligence quotients and uses this as a basis to inspire individuals to reach a higher level of control of their abilities. Most of the time we think something and then perform in a different way, which is usually due to the confusion between our thoughts and our actions. NLP aids in reducing the dissonance that exists between our thinking processes and actions. It creates a more coherence between our thoughts and beliefs and the actions we take. It also helps stabilize the thinking process and allows us make more considered choices, even in the midst in the heat of the moment. It aids us in seeing the bigger picture, increasing our capacity to collect the wealth of information that comes into the process of making decisions, thereby providing an enhanced perspectives. NLP is designed to assist us in to better manage all the information that we receive to make a decision.

Parameters

NLP is currently being used across a range of fields including sales, psychology healthcare, and even businesses. The use to NLP in any field is governed by the following factors.

Neurological

Our nervous system is comprised of two essential parts, namely the peripheral nervous system (which is responsible for our reflexes) and the central nervous system (rational thinking that accompanies actions). The way in which the central nervous system assists us to react to different circumstances is completely dependent on the way we perceive. NLP is a method of altering our perception in an approach that helps individuals to develop more effective, constructive responses due to fundamental changes in the way we view things and comprehend them.

Linguistic

Language is often an obstacle to communicating our thoughts. Since our choices are mostly dependent on our internal conversations It is essential to communicate these thoughts properly and concisely after they have been released to the world. A clear and concise message can not only reduce confusion but also aid us in our efforts to reach our goals of perfection. NLP is designed to assist us to reorganize our internal dialogue and flow from a different viewpoint and an interpretative framework.

Programming

NLP is accomplished by synchronizing the thoughts and language. An organized mind is crucial to take the right decisions and implementing the results. The ability to program our minds can enable us to distinguish emotions when making decisions. This will prevent irrationality, confusion and impulsivity that can be caused by a poorly thought-out emotional responses.

Mind levels

This is the last factor that is the final parameter in NLP. The three levels of our minds, specifically subconscious (responsible in interpreting intuition) and the subconscious (consists of available but not clearly defined information) and the conscious (state of consciousness) are the ones responsible for the operation that our brains perform. NLP seeks to access the information that is stored in our subconscious mind due to past experiences and making it available for the interpretation of your conscious brain. This gives us access to more options for knowledge and action, since we are able to "get at" details that we might otherwise be unnoticed as having.

How do they work?

NLP is based on modalities which are representations of our various experiences. The modalities are further separated into submodalities (perceptions stemming out of our sensory senses smell, touch, and vision). NLP attempts to accomplish the desired result by altering the submodalities. These modifications alter the original experience and then replace it. The actions we take are therefore altered in accordance with the altered experience.

Let's look at the various aspects of NLP:

It is important to understand your actions. Because NLP is designed to alter your thinking and actions it is crucial to be aware of your behavior first. Be aware of how you respond to different situations , and take note of these. By observing your reactions over time you'll be able identify the pattern of your actions, and help to identify submodalities.

After you are in a position to discern your reactions to various situations, what should be done is to determine how they could be modified to achieve the desired results and to create a more efficient communication with other people. To do this it is necessary to be aware of how others react to similar situations. Compare your reactions to other people's and then analyze. Take note of areas where you could improve.

Once you have analyzed your actions and identified areas that could be improved Now, you must apply this knowledge to change your behaviour. Make an outline of goals to be associated with the desired behavior change. The goal-setting process will help you feel in direction, and can aid in the process of programming your brain.

Once you've got your list of goals, the next thing to be addressed is forming your action plans. Develop a strategy in response to your observations of your behaviour. This is what makes your plan distinct. Each plan is unique because no two are alike because people don't behave in exactly the same way. It is important to ensure that your plan includes your areas of improvement that you've noted.

When you begin using the NLP plan, be aware of your improvements. Examine how you've progressed in each submodality. Don't lose hope even if you do not attain the desired outcomes in the initial phase of implementation. Very few individuals achieve success in the initial phase. Keep track of your failures and also your accomplishments. This will allow you to identify other weaknesses in your actions, that didn't come up during the initial observation phase. Continue to refine your strategy, taking into account what might not have been successful

during the initial phase of implementation.
Be sure to thank yourself for any small
victories you might achieve in the process
of implementation. This can keep you
motivated to continue following the plan
in the long run.

O The final stage of NLP is to formulate an
action plan that should not be rigid in its
implementation and allow you to alter it in
line with the information you've learned.
When you are preparing an idea, it's
crucial that you don't set unreliable
expectations for its execution. Since it's
not possible to anticipate every possible
obstacle or delay There must be some
degree of flexibility within your plan.
Consider ways to modify your existing plan
to be flexible and flexible, in order to
adapt to changes you may have to make. It
is important to ensure that your plan is in
place continuously. You might be required
to make changes to your current plan to
accomplish this. Be careful not to
complicate your strategy by adding more

steps. It could make it difficult to follow through with. Each step requires your attention and effort Be conscious of this when planning.

For NLP to be effective, you should be willing to look at your perceptions and responses honestly and systematically, as well as hold them up against exemplary examples of similar perceptive-responsive models. By learning to understand your own perceptions as well as the responses that result from them, you will be more effective at engaging others and avoiding emotional interference that could cause harm to your relationships and others' perceptions of your character. Through deconstructing your thinking and emotional processes and changing how you decide to choose the words you speak and act you'll discover that you'll soon be modeling the behavior that distinguishes you as an outstanding example. It is essential to remain committed towards the endeavor and ready to dedicate the time needed to ensure it works for you.

Chapter 11: Putting The End To The Show In Safety

.All your skits are over and your audience has been entertained. What do you have to do is to snap your fingers to awake the 'victims then pack up and go to your home? NO!

These volunteers have been your lifeline, and you've earned a paycheck every night. You must do more for them prior to they leave on their way. One thing that should be mentioned during the introduction (as also) is that when they quit the auditorium (hall or theatre, gymnasium whatever venue you're using for the performance) for longer than five minutes, any prior or post suggestions to hypnotize them that you've provided them with are instantly cancelled and they'll be alert and awake. This protects them in the event that they were hypnotized to react in a particular manner to triggers. Dancing like Elvis could be hilarious on stage, but what could occur if someone was driving and heard the exact Elvis track? (Chances are that nothing will happen. The mind's instinct to protect itself will override your idea But why risk it?).

When you have them come out of their trance use the moment to throw some positive affirmations. Let them know that they've experienced the best moment of their lives They have an uncluttered mind and are going to return home to the most restful sleep of their lives and wake up feeling fantastic. One of the most effective and most convincing ways to inform them is that they'll never remember anything about the main entertainer in that night (hypnotic amnesia). Your guests will enjoy some laughs, and will be even more convinced about your magical abilities which is benefit for your next trip to the region. They will also be convinced of the need to purchase the DVD you'll be selling from the evening's show to ensure they can remember what they saw even if they don't remember the event. (See the next chapter for Making a Bit Extra on the next page).

However, even if you've instructed them to "One Three, Two, Three. Wide Awake" They'll seem quite charming for a couple of minutes afterward make sure to keep the positive messages , and steer clear of the possibility of making any negative suggestion or chance of someone in their vicinity making any suggestions. It is usually performed by asking for another applause for the participants before they go back into their seating. This is one of the rounds that you ought to make sure you milk for your guests and keep them on the air for hours... even if they don't know the reason!

British Law and common sense suggests it. You probably will in the end to clean the props and equipment, however, you should stay for at minimum half an hour following the show in case there are any small issues they have to take care of. We're not advocating therapy, however one of the physiological effects that come with Trance (and which is meditation as well as the hypnotic state) could be headaches due to dehydration. Drinking a glass of water slowly is the best cure and your thoughtful attitude will be noticed. A second tick for future appointments.

If you're a local and offer hypnotherapy there is a chance that you will get more appointments for those who want to quit smoking, shed excess weight, get rid of fears and other issues that are typical of therapy. Avoid therapy sessions after the show. Your 'customers' and neither you are in a positive mindset, but don't be afraid of asking for a booking of a therapy session or even provide a business card and of course, use separate cards for shows and therapy aspects of your hypnosis sessions.

If you're outside the city and you don't have access to a therapy CDs on your Back of Room (BoR) tables for sales even if they're not the ones you are using for therapy. Some stage hypnotists earn substantial income through BoR. Why should you be different?

Another tip is that when you know that you'll be going to return to this venue or another nearby venue, make sure that your participants receive free tickets. This could be due to either of the two motives. One reason is that they didn't see the show because they were in it, and more importantly, they don't even remember being a part of the show (because YOU told them to forget everything) This is why they may are eager to see the show again. Another reason is because YOU advised them to enjoy the show, so they might like to experience the same hypnotism again. You now have a quick completely compliant and dependable volunteer. The perfect superstar for your next production. A the hypno-junkie. SCORE!

Making A Bit Extra - Sales & Publicity

Commonly referred to commonly as BoR or "back of room" the sales could increase the earnings you earn during your evening. DVDs of shows from the past (or even that particular evening's performance when you're organised) will always be a big hit and, if you've got a thoughts of therapy (or even in the absence of any) self-hypnosis CDs that address common ailments like weight loss and quitting smoking, anxiety of flying, and the improvement of self-confidence and study skills can also be a good seller. If you're not interested in creating your own therapy CDs you can hire a hypnotherapist record your recordings in exchange for a portion of profits or for an unbeatable fee.

DVDs and CDs must have professional printing, framed and packaged with a custom case with your information even if it's not your voice that is being used. Your actions as well as your image, which these purchases are constructed on.

They aren't usually an effective seller, however you can have a giveaway page (professionally made with your personal name web address and contact information if you'd like to get more bookings) which includes your book's title (or an alternative's if you aren't writing any yet) available on Amazon, Smashwords, Lulu and so on. (try to mail them through your website. Then, you can make the links to your products connected and receive a larger revenue from them should they buy something else from the sales website).

Be sure that everything you offer or sell is clearly branded by your name, your website and contact information - a paper label, if anything, however professionally printed is superior. In the end , it's the only way to promote your business.

126

The key is if you have the opportunity to earn extra dollars, pounds or shekels in the currencies of your choice and you are able to, then do. Make use of your fame while you have it, but it might just last for the duration of the evening.

What else do you need?

The next paragraphs provide a list things to consider regarding the location, your safety and the safety of the participants, people who attend the venue. Thanks for Jonathan Royle (UK based hypnotist and trainer) for helping me become conscious of the significance of these issues.

You've been scheduled to appear at a place and it's your first visit there. It is important to be aware of the following.

Are the stages smooth? Wearing carpets or edges that have been lifted can be a danger to walk on.

Do you have anything stuck up that could cause a accident or fall? Do you have your hypnotes away from lighting fixtures and speakers?

Do you know of a method that allows you to create an appropriate safety line away from any stage? A white piece of tape works the best option for this scenario. Remember that you have to tell your participants not to overstep the white line while they are performing on the stage. Be sure that your marks aren't in direct contact with edge of the stage space.

Is there a secure method for your guests to get on and off the stage without disturbing the crowd? The steps that climb steeply should be secured with safety rails or staff on the stage to assist volunteers.

Are the chairs sturdy? Chairs that fold can be an injury risk.

There could be other aspects you should take into consideration. Do you have trained staff or do you depend on the staff at the venue? If you're the latter, then you'll need to train them on the duties they are expected to perform. It is better to train your own assistants and let the venue staff to lead the performers onto the stage, to your kind kindnesses.

In all places, barring the most modest venues, you'll require a sound system or at least one type. You could decide to purchase one yourself or hire it as needed. If you're organized, you'll make the purchase of sound systems a part of the contract, however you'll still require the dimensions of your venue to determine the power of the amplifier and speaker systems needed.

One thing you must always be equipped with is your own microphone(s). According to your local radio regulations and regulations, you must be equipped with at least a UHF (not VHF - they are more susceptible to interference) microphone or two. If you choose to use headset, hand-held mic, or Lavalier (tie pin clip) design is dependent on the way you plan to communicate with your participants. It is not possible to hand them headset microphones to them, nor do you take the time to wire them individually, so a handheld microphone that you can hold and point at them is generally the best choice. Or, headsets or Lavalier for you , and an ample pouch or holster for the mic you have in your hand those times you require both hands.

A variety of spares including batteries, are crucial and having an backup plan in case of emergency, a corded mic and extension leads that are long may help you avoid the worst. Don't be stingy with this equipment.

The amount you spend on hardware is entirely up to you. You decide how much you consider stage work to be your profession as well as how professionally you wish to appear.

There are a lot of stage hypnotists that bring 1or 2 digital video cameras to capture as many of their performances as they can. Some bring computers as well as multi-DVD burning equipment, to allow the audience to take home a DVD of the show. The more equipment you have and the more people you'll need, and they'll all want to be compensated for sacrificing their night. An entourage can cost you money, but you can't manage it all on your own.

From a security point of standpoint as well as a marketing one, recording each show is vital. However, how you approach in the future is your choice. Videos to be used on websites, YouTube and promotional material is considered essential for every entertainer today.

The most important thing to remember is that no matter what equipment you have, make sure to practice using it. If you're all thumbs and fingers with an instrument that you hold, it will be obvious to your audience and even the other volunteers. If you don't have an idea of how to set the entire thing up before getting started, you'll appear like an amateur. Learn your craft. Everything.

Chapter 12: Power of Self-hypnosis

We can begin using hypnosis for yourself first. Self-hypnosis is an enjoyable, relaxing experience. It can assist you relax and relieve tension. It's a kind of meditation that permits you to communicate with yourself. It's a means to relax and forget your worries for a few minutes.

Self-hypnosis is a great way to increase your ability to learn, improve memories, and remain aware during an exam or important workplace presentation. It is a great tool to hold your hand in case you're facing the stress of an emotionally exhausting event. It will assist you in clearing the clutter out of your head following a hectic agenda.

When practiced often over the long run Self-hypnosis can eventually become your lifestyle as a regular, exclusive time for you. It could lead one to greater understanding of your own self and other people. It could also alter how you lead in your daily life, think about your choices or manage relationships.

Self-hypnosis can help you slow down and breathe completely. It is often the most basic of items like these get overlooked in our busy lives. The steps to self-hypnosis are really quite easy. Gather yourself locate a quiet spot to concentrate, and all else will come after. However, once you've been tasked with doing it, we may find the simple task of settling down (being at a halt for few minutes) quite difficult. In our busy, short-attention span society, sitting still and unoccupied is a challenge in itself. However, once you do it, everything else will come naturally.

Let's test some self-hypnosis exercises using a few factors required to run a successful hypnosis session.

Quiet Time

If you're sharing a home with others, choose an appointment time where there are less activities that can distract you. If you're living on your own make sure you do it at a time in the time you're least expecting people to stop by, phone or text you. It's better to switch off your mobile.

You'll have a Room of Your Own

Find a peaceful spot far from the bustle and noise of the home. You should ensure that the environment is calm and suitable for self-hypnosis. Turn off the light, flicker several candles and sprinkle some incense if you want. Set the temperature of the room in accordance with your preferences.

Reclining or sitting in a comfy spot. Relax with cushions and pillows. Be sure that you are at ease, so that you are able to stay in the position for a long time.

Include Nature Sounds or Music

In movies, like in real life, music can set the mood for every kind of scene. Play some relaxing music in the player. Relaxing music can have different meanings to individuals. It's all about personal preferences Hardcore metal might seem "comforting" to certain people (maybe it brings him back to high school) However, it's not suitable for the self-hypnosis sessions that we envision. Try this switch on the music and notice your heartbeat. If it encourages or maintains the pace of a slow rhythm, that's great. The sounds of nature can be very effective like ocean waves and the whistling wind, the ringing of the chimes sound of leaves rustling, or the soft gurgle of the water brook. If your home has a tiny desk fountain, set it in close proximity to where your. Keep in mind how the sound from water always soothes.

An Awhiff Of Memory

The olfactory nerves are the first ones to develop after birth and the only one to remain with us after we pass away. The work of a Nobel Peace Prize winner discusses the fact that the sense of smell is an essential and crucial element in our memory. The research shows how much we are able to remember simply by recalling certain scents, and the ways that this ability has assisted the survival of humans and their development since.

Did you notice how the smell of certain substances can greatly affect our emotions more than other sense? The smell of a scent can alter our mood, transport us back in time or remind us of the special person in our lives. Mothers might have the sharpest sense of smell studies have shown that they can discern their children even the grown-ups through their distinct smells.

However, we can also increase our relaxation simply by playing with our sense of scent. Prior to your exercise, it is possible to soak in a tub as well as wash and dry your hair with the most deliciously scented shampoo and soap. It is possible to massage aromatherapy oil onto your skin. Burn aromatherapy candles or oil. Incense is a great way to light. Your body and your mind will respond positively to these pleasures. If the hypnosis session you are having might not succeed, you will at least are smelling and feeling well.

Feel It

As a few of us be able to sense smell, there are some who are kinesthetic. That is they react strongly to the touch. They are attracted to being at ease and touch others. They enjoy the feeling of soft, silky material in their hands. They like to rub their fingers over an interestingly rough surface. They will often hug someone or pat their backs and in return , they want to do the same to themselves.

If you're one of the people who are in that category, benefit from it to increase your level of relaxation. Relax in a comfortable bed with cushions. Feel the silky feel of sheets for your bed. Dress in your most soft and comfortable clothing. Massage some moisturizing lotion onto your skin, and allow your hands to feel relax. Feel the breeze as it moves and gets into your skin and hair.

The Self-Hypnosis The Script

Hypnosis's power as we've seen lies in the ability to suggest. The key to a successful suggestion is selecting the appropriate words, expressing them in the correct way and at the appropriate timing. It is essential to be completely convincing, but you should not be imploring. Be firm, but not overly insistent. Soft, but not weak. Of course, a lot of this is dependent on your words and how you express it.

Below is an example self-hypnosis script. The most common hypnosis scripts comprise three primary components: the introduction along with the suggestions, and the end which can differ greatly in content and technique. The induction triggers the hypnosis process and allows you relax your entire body and eliminate stress. If you can relax your body, you will be able to improve your quality of life in all aspects physically, mentally emotionally, spiritually, and physically.

The suggestions section of a typical script in which you include positive remarks about what you would like to work on or improve.

The end is when you begin the count until fully alertness.

The following script contains an introduction and a conclusion. It is possible to make suggestions according to your own preferences. It is recommended to record and tape the entire script, then play it in your session.

The SCRIPT'S FIRST LINES

Place a candle in the light and put it before you, in a position where you can view the flame from an ideal angle.

Find a comfortable seating position. Set yourself up with blankets and pillows If you have to.

The soft glowing light Watch it dance and swing slowly, slowly in a peaceful way, like you are at the moment. (Pause)

Breathe in, breathe out. Breathe in through your nose and lightly blow air from your slightly opened mouth. (Pause)

Breathe in, exhale out. (Pause)

Repeat. Breathe in, breathe out. Breathe in and out. (Pause) Breathe deeply and breathe the breath of fresh breath into healthy lung. Feel it filled with fresh, sweet air. (Pause)

Inhale and let all your tension out of your body. (Pause) Breathe. Relax. As relaxed and tranquil as the flickering fire in front of you. (Pause)

The flame is soft. The light of the flame is yellow as the stars are, when you're asleep. The flame is warm to your eyes. You can feel them closing slowly. (Pause)

The eyes have become tired and they are weighing down. Your eyes are beginning to close. You're tempted to shut your eyes tight. (Pause)

Your eyes remain warm. The warmth of the flame around them. Even with your eyes closed you can clearly see the flame dancing ahead of you. (Pause)

In and out you breathe. When you take a deeper breath and relax, the more at peace, and very deeply now. (Pause)

The warmth radiates across your face. The warmth is all over. (Pause)

Your forehead is glowing. A bright, light and bright light shines off your forehead. (Pause)

The soft, warm light is spread across your face. You face relaxes. Relaxing more and more. (Pause)

Inhaling and exhaling, you feel more relaxed. out, you'll feel more at ease than ever before. (Pause)

You breathe, and you feel your chest full of air. The air is warm. The light of your face reaches your neck and down to your chest. (Pause)

Breathe in deeply now. The soft, warm light soothes your body and as comfortable and slack as the skin. (Pause)

The soft, warm and relaxing light is spread across your arms, your hands, and even to even the ends of your fingers. You feel so calm now. (Pause)

The soft, warm and relaxing light is spread into your stomach, up to your waist, and finally to your hips. You're feeling so relaxed. (Pause)

The soft, warm and relaxing light stretches further towards your back. Your back is so relaxed today. (Pause)

Your breathing is slow and deep both in and out. You are more than ever are feeling so calm and relaxed. (Pause)

The soft, warm and relaxing light stretches into your thighs and down to your legs. It's like they're relaxed. The weight that is placed on them is slowly becoming as if it's light. (Pause)

It's like you're in a state of relaxation. Every muscle, each tissue inside your body feels smooth. You feel so peaceful. (Pause)

You breathe in and breathe out. You go deeper and deeper into relaxation. (Pause)

The soft, warm gentle light stretches to your feet up to the tips of your toes. The feet feel so comfortable today. Everything that's put on them gradually feels like a breeze. (Pause)

Imagine yourself standing on the most soft, green grass you've ever put your feet on. Your feet are very soft and warm. (Pause) You're in a field that is open. The sun is warm and it is a pleasure to be around you. (Pause)

A cool breeze blows across your locks, body, and even your face. It moves across the grassy field combing every delicate green tiny sliver. (Pause)

You stroll through the fields of soft warm grass. You can see a mountain far away. You slowly stroll toward the mountain. (Pause)

As you stroll towards the blue, warm mountain, you sink further and farther into a state of relaxation. Your body is so calm and relaxed. (Pause)

Your mind is alert and sharp you are able to process every aspect in perfect. (Pause)

In perfect harmony, just like the small stream that you see while traveling. The sound of the stream soothes you more than you can imagine. You walk along the tiny stream, and your feet are getting wet from the clear, warm water. The water is more relaxing than ever. (Pause)

You'll walk more and more, towards the mountains. (Pause)

A soft, warm breeze blows through you combing your hair, going through your clothes, your body. Then, slowly, gradually lifting you like an airborne feather. (Pause)

The wind lifts you , and you feel as if you are floating in the soft, sweet air. You are weightless as you sink deeper into a state of relaxation. (Pause)

The climb continues to get higher until you finally reach the summit on the mountain. (Pause)

There are a few small wildflowers at the top on the mountains. They are a wonderful fresh, clean scent. You inhale the lovely fresh, clean scent of the mountain air. (Pause)

The wind gradually, slowly, takes you lower down the mountain. As you descend lower and lower, you become more conscious. Each time you count, you begin to slowly come out of your deep sleep. (Pause)

[End of Induction[End of Induction

Add any suggestions you have here[Begin Ending[Begin Conclusion

Each time you listen this recording for self-hypnosis you'll get deeper, more calm, and reap greater benefits from the experience. (Pause)

One...

The scent of the soft fresh rain is within you. It's in your hair, on your hands, and your body. It's like rain. The scent is of optimism, of the creation process and of renewed life.

Two...

Lower your feet, down into the grassy field. Lower until your feet are in the soft, warm grass again.

Three...

At the rate of five, you'll be more awake, vibrant and energized than you have ever been.

Four...

Remember the aroma of rain? It gives the new season, new hopes.

Five. Refreshed, awake, and fully prepared! End of SCRIPT

Do this regularly. You'll be amazed at how effective it is.

Chapter 13: The Truth Concerning Hypnosis and Covert Hypnosis

What is the main difference between normal hypnosis and the covert hypnosis?

It allows you to influence people to perform exactly the way you want them accomplish in almost any situation. To induce a person into the state of hypnosis, an induction process is employed during regular hypnosis. A part of the brain is shut down, also called the critical factor in the process of induction. Usually, the critical factor determines the suggestions that are accepted by the unconscious mind.

The critical element can reject suggestions that do not agree with the ones accepted in the normal state of consciousness. But, the critical factor is not activated while a person is under an hypnotic state and it's easy for suggestions to be absorbed into the subconscious mind.

This is processed if it's true, once suggestions are accepted into unconscious mind. To get around the crucial factor the use of specific language patterns to induce hypnosis covertly. In the absence of induction, these patterns allow suggestions to gain into unconscious mind. That means that during the course of a conversation, you can instruct the person to obey an instruction.

During sales presentations, occult hypnosis is a popular technique due to obvious motives. Most often, salespeople use it.

To convey one meaning for your subconscious, and another to your conscious brain the use of uncertain words often. Perhaps "By today" is the most popular phrase' among these.

In the final moments of a presentation , the "By now" method is often used. It sounds like a joke.

Infused into any presentation, the ambiguity of the word "by" lets be the (rather simple) enclosed request "Buy Right Now".

Imagine that you're carrying a pencil. If you wish to, you can break the pencil with ease. Breaking the pencil is a sign of the ability to defy covert hypnosis.

It is easy to break two or three pencils. However, it is somewhat difficult to break four or five pencils. It becomes difficult breaking eight of them.

It's similar to adding a pencil each time a hypnotist adds an additional covert instance in the course of conversation. It's surprising to realize how powerful covert hypnosis can be when you think about how one sentence can easily contain up and five patterns of covert hypnosis.

Imagine, in an ordinary conversation in the bar or during an upcoming sales presentation, think of how many hidden patterns you might cover.

You could be surprised by this fact. It's easy to get someone to become enthralled with you using hypnosis covert. For seduction only it is possible to find a number of specially made covert hypnosis patterns are out there. It is essential to be capable of backing it up when you attempt to lure someone with the use of covert techniques of hypnosis.

To make someone become a fan of it is possible to use covert hypnosis. Your life could be altered by hypnosis covertly, in the event that you're an average guy who is shy and aren't sure how to get women to talk to you. Don't expect anything to be the case if you're an unrepentant jerk who wants to use hypnosis covertly to make a hole in the bedpost. In order to make someone feel attracted to your personality, you only need to make a subtle gesture towards yourself, such as at certain times, and then rub your chest. In a normal conversation, using this method is thought to be the best method to make a connection with a friend. It is important to determine what character traits you admire of the person you're going to influence. When you say something that's connected to these characteristics, simply make a gesture towards yourself.

For example, when you hear terms like romance, passion, exhilarating or sexually attractive, you could want to make a gesture to yourself.

Most likely, you'd perform this action instinctively if you tried to convey your name to a stranger. Someone else would instantly be able to understand if you made a gesture towards yourself when you say your name. The subconscious brain interprets the gesture as meaning that this is who I am, and this is who I am. Certain words are associated with your body when you make gestures towards yourself based on them.

If you'd like your chance of receiving a boost in your pay make sure you use words such as reliable, hardworking or reliable every when you are having a conversation in front of your manager.

"A majority people consider sales and seduction as the primary two areas, however, covert hypnosis could be utilized for a whole lot more".

If you know what it can do such as avoiding fines, being exempted from tickets, avoiding the lines, obtaining free upgrades, or simply making your kids do their homework is easy.

Chapter 14: Instructional Guidelines and The Self-Hypnosis scripts

Self-hypnosis offers a way to help you reach the subconscious mind. It is possible to study hypnosis, and then apply it to yourself to make modifications in your personality. Because it works through the subliminal sphere that can alter the patterns of actuation and rationality in their source. The changes could persist for the duration of a lifetime.

There are a variety of methods for self-hypnosis, however they all begin with the same initial action by putting yourself in a relaxed at ease and open mental state. If your mind is in a state of relaxation, you will have direct access to your subconscious, where the patterns of your thinking and behavior are stored.

Inhaling deeply is essential in achieving your state that you want. It is, however, a matter of practice and consistent use. You'll likely be surprised to find out that lots of people do not understand how to breathe properly. Every breath should be regular and prolonged.

It is recommended not to overdo your breathing. While practicing, you can take note of your breaths get in a minute. Begin with one breath all the way up to 25. If you're not at a level of calm then count until you are at one. By doing this, you can take your mind off worries and help you focus on breathing.

You can then go on to visualizing. This is the process to reflect on where your peaceful spot is. It could be the white, sand beach, a lush mountain lea that is surrounded by lush green or an emerald-colored forest or on a boat within the ocean's vast blue. Think of any location that will provide you with a feeling of calm, and put yourself there in your thoughts.

After imagining yourself in the setting you prefer You can now apply auto-suggestive methods. The most straightforward method to self-hypnosis is to use affirmative statements. These are simple phrases or words which you repeat to yourself in the state of hypnosis.

Slowly as you repeat that mantra it'll become written in your subconscious mind. The lines could be any thing, but they must be positive and positive. Your subconscious mind reacts strongly to negative statements and will certainly dismiss them.

Positive affirmations employ words to alter your subconscious mind. When you imagine the image inside your brain, it is likely that you will be achieving whatever you wish to accomplish. If you're looking to beat an illness, picture you are healthy. If you're using self-hypnosis techniques to enhance your writing abilities, imagine your name being mentioned as an the author of a book. If financial success is what you desire then train your brain to visualize yourself as the president and CEO of a huge business empire. The self-hypnosis methods focus on positive thoughts. Similar to mantras, negative images should not be employed.

It is crucial to close the hypnotic session with a uplifting image. Being a novice it is crucial to devise a strategy to end a session correctly. Although there is no danger of being trapped in a hypnotized state , and not being able to return to normal life, it could be unpleasant if done correctly, and this potentially dangerous event may reduce its effectiveness.

The ideal way to return to reality is to be relaxed, slow and steady. This should always be a procedure that you perform the same way each time. The most effective method is a simple reversal of the self-hypnosis method you utilized to reach the hypnotic state.

For instance, if you notice yourself heading down a staircase, you can see yourself walking slowly back up the staircase. Anyone can hypnotize. It is common to see hypnosis performed on stage performed by people we think of being able to do magic. However, this is not the case.

Anyone can hypnotize themselves by consistently studying and gaining experience with the techniques. Training is the most crucial component of self-hypnosis. Most techniques appear quite simple at first. But, once you get started making it happen, you'll realize how difficult it is.

The ability to put yourself in a serene state is more complicated than most people realize. By constant and constant practice , however, you will improve your self-hypnosis techniques easily. Once you have mastered the art of hypnosis, it might be beneficial to try it with other people.

Hypnotizing others is known as "hetero-hypnosis." The two methods are fundamentally the same. One thing which is the difference is that with self-hypnosis techniques, you are employing them on yourself with anyone else helping you.

When you finally choose to learn the skills and expertise of hypnosis be aware that it takes lots of time to learn and master. You'll need to stay persistent and committed without any expectation that it will happen instantly.

It usually requires quite a few trials before self-hypnosis methods start to yield results. When you learn to better and more successfully manage your mind, it will be much easier to enter the state of hypnosis and to alter the subconscious mind.

Self-hypnosis is a method of self-hypnosis that can be utilized to help you with a myriad of motives. Here are some scripts and images you can explore for each purpose:

1. Stop the habit of smoking

Image: You can see your reflection in a mirror. You notice that you have wrinkles and lines that are less prominent on your face. Your lips have slowly turned pink and your teeth became white. Your breath has changed to sweet and sweet-smelling, and you no more have pimples around your mouth.

The script reads: "I am more beautiful and youthful looking due to the fact that I haven't smoked anymore."

2. To manage anger

Image: You're looking through the paper for the day while sipping a hot cup freshly brewed coffee in the office. You're waiting on the late reports of your subordinates before you begin your portion of the job. You're confident in the knowledge that even should they have to submit the report at lunchtime it will still be completed it on time.

Text: "I am too competent and talented to be influenced by the incompetence of other people. I can work more quickly than others and I still have enough time to finish the report in the time frame."

3. For managing stress and anxiety.

Image: You can see yourself singing along as you cook for the holiday family dinner.You are dressed to impress and well-groomed. Your apron is even coordinating with the colour of your gown. You've cooked a meal for your kids and their family members who will be coming within a couple of minutes.

Text: "I am proud of my loving and successful children. Together, they and their parents and spouse will relish the dinner I carefully selected to serve tonight."

4. To enhance self-confidence

Image: You're on a stage receiving a glass platter to acknowledge the remarkable contribution you've made for the business you work with. The ceremony is a formal dinner held at an elite hotel located in the center of the city. You also got a job promotion, and your husband who took you to the event, beams with pride , as do the crowd who are clapping in a standing ovations.

The script: "I can do excellent work since I'm satisfied doing it. I am able to do better as it keeps my husband feel proud and happy about me being his wife."

5. to improve your appearance

Image The couple are attending a gala celebration of the company. The ballroom is packed with colleagues from the workplace and spouses. You are beaming with joy as the women are looking at you with a second glance of your adoring husband. Your husband seems to be unaware of all the ladies around him since his attention is on you and your radiant beauty.

Text: "I am the luckiest girl alive to be and loved by my beloved husband. He chose me ahead of other women and I will make his decision a good one."

6. To enhance creativity

Image: You're signing your books that became bestsellers. There is a crowds of people waiting to get your signature following the purchase of an edition. The publisher of your book is thrilled and satisfied. He's busy making plans for the next book's launch.

The script reads: "I can and will create a book that is of immense value to many people. They will buy the books I write because they were written to assist them."

7. To develop spirituality

Image: You're walking by yourself on a beach. You notice another footprints that were walking along with you, but and there is no one else. You feel a sense of peace and security in the knowledge that you're not the only one and will never be while walking. You begin to talk to this unnoticed friend, and the breeze responds to you with songs.

The script reads: "My God will always be with me wherever I go and in whatever I do. I may not be able to see Him But He'll be with me in every step I make in my life."

8. To develop a correct sleeping routine

Image: You're lying on a hammock securely tucked to two coconuts in a picturesque location near to the ocean. It is clear to see the blue skies and soft white clouds. When you close your eyes you can hear soft whispers from the wind and the soft strokes of the waves along the shore.

The script reads: "I will sleep peacefully being surrounded by the beauty of nature. Nothing in the world that could deprive me of this rest."

Chapter 15: What to Inspiring Strangers to Hypnotize

The act of hypnotizing a stranger or someone who you've had a brief conversation with but haven't really spoken to can be a challenge when compared against the ease with which you can hypnotize someone who you are familiar with. The problem lies in the fact that it's more difficult to convince someone who is a stranger or who you don't know to let you hypnotize them.

How to Impress Strangers Social Gatherings

But, there's an easy method to charm strangers.

Step 1

If you're at a party where you would like to make someone hypnotize you or see whether a person will heed your instructions, sit on the wall or a chair and look around the crowd. Find someone who you think has a lot of charm and be willing to be hypnotized and listen to your instructions. For the beginning it is recommended to pick a target that is easy to reach.

Step 2

If you come across a fascinating subject, talk to him/her in a friendly manner, and then enter the circle the person is standing in.

The first thing to do is to establish a good relationships with the person. To achieve this, keep close eye contact with the person, and smile at that person several times. Pay attention to the person closely and note any noticeable body or gesture that they make regularly. If your subject is known to regularly run the fingers of his or hers through the hair of theirs or shakes constantly his or her leg, watch it and then try to mimic the gesture. This is referred to"mirroring.'

Mirroring is an effective method that allows you to capture your target's attention and build relationships with them at a subconscious level. In this way, the person will feel attracted to you , and you'll find an easier way to affect them.

Step 3.

Begin to talk to him/her through small talk, and gradually build it up. When you're sure the person is more at ease with you, ask them what they would like to learn an act of kindness. Most people answer to this question with a "yes"; it is very likely that the person you're trying to influence to say that too.

Step 4

Then, you can hypnotize the person by using the techniques you learned from the last chapter. If putting someone to sleep is a challenge you can say things like as "You are doing well. Be calm and relaxed like you do when you are sleeping."

By using your hands, you can guide your subject's gaze downwards when you speak. Use suggestions such as "you wouldn't wish that to happen, wouldn't you?' The subconscious removes negative words, such as "not" from suggestions and then alters the phrases. If you remove the word 'not' from the above suggestion the suggestion becomes "You would prefer that that occur, right?" This way, the subject will concentrate on sleep and soon be in a state of trance.

Step 5

When your subject gets slouched over and falls on you, allow him/her to lay on your shoulders and assist in calming him/her. Make sure to place him/her in a comfortable chair so that when he/she awakes the next morning, you will know that you put him/her in an armchair and did not make any kind of profit of them.

170

Then, you can talk to the person about what you'd like to talk about and ask questions that you'd like to ask. To stimulate your subject follow the same procedure that were discussed in the previous chapter.

Like everything else, the best method to master this technique is to practice it as frequently as you can. Once you are able to master the art of hypnosis, you'll achieve great strength and employ it in a variety of circumstances to manipulate and control individuals.

If, for instance, you master the art of hypnotizing people, you will not allow your boss to treat you badly or let your colleagues ridicule your every day. You will also be an effective speaker and develop the capacity to utilize your words to persuade and influence others. Most of the time it is not possible to hypnotize people by putting them into the state of trance immediately. But, you can do it by using words. Thus, try practicing hypnosis in a covert manner whenever you can since you'll use it often.

Chapter 16: Effortless Relationship that creates a deep connection

If you are trying to convince someone, you need to make them agree with you. It's not necessary to, but it's definitely more effective this method.

Rapport is the feeling of connection between two people when your focus is directed towards one another and you feel like you're on the same page.'

Change-making meetings in which changes occur are triggered by the relationship.

You've had this type of relationships numerous times in the past as you've been talking with friends and having a good time, or engaging in a great lengthy conversation.

Rapport isn't just a one-on-one the other hand; a professional speaker is able to connect with the audience. That is the best speaker gets in conversation with their audience.

How do we come up with the "rapport?"

In the beginning of this book, I spoke at length with you concerning NLP. NLP is the method of modeling effective behaviours in order to develop techniques and patterns is a big deal when it comes to rapport.

The issue is that I think they made a mistake.

They say that in order to build relationship with people, you should match and reflect.

You mimic subtly your body expressions, gestures and language to make it appear the impression that you are both alike.

NLP is a plethora of techniques to help make this process more subtle yet at its most fundamental level , that's what it boils down to.

How did NLP arrive at the conclusion that re-enacting gestures is the primary factor for efficient communication?

Simple as that: They watched. You can go to a cafe, bar or coffee shop, and then watch the crowd at work.

Check out the intimate couples, as well as the friends who are laughing and watch the body expressions.

They usually have the same posture or sitting in the same way. This is a wonderful observation, but it does not necessarily work in reverse.

Being in rapport could make you mirror your body language however, mirroring one another's body language will not always result in you being in contact.

It's as if rich people have a lot of money. Therefore in order to become wealthy, you must invest a lot of money!

Let's give NLP its proper due, there's some logic behind mirroring and matching body language.

The fact is that physiology does influence the state of mind.

Lean back in your chair right now Smile and relax.

Relax and smile in that posture at least 30 seconds trying to make it appear as real as is possible.

It's likely that you'll start to feel better because of it? Your body is triggering the physiological connections to happiness.

But, real happiness is a result of more than altering your posture.

True rapport is also caused by many more things other than simply altering how you speak!

* A note for angry NLPers: Those who are sensible will not believe the flood of angry emails that I receive when I debunk the

NLP myth. It is likely that this book will provoke some.

Good. You purchased this product to discover new things, right? Therefore, I'd be doing you an injustice if I kept to the traditional ideas and taught just like all the other students.

Take this book with an open heart, and If it challenges your views it's fine! Learning is about embracing new ideas, but it would be a bit naive to claim that everything in this book was a gospel. At this point, you can try the book and see if you can use these concepts and techniques work for you.

How to Create Really Good Rapport

Now I've shattered the myth on the traditional matching or mirroring myths, we can take a look at how you can actually build an effective relationship.

It's really time to return to the basics.

Dale Carnegie (author of "How to Make Friends, Influence and Win the Love of People") basic.

Rapport is a way to connect Therefore, don't waste time thinking about fancy methods and just go out and begin connecting!

The main thing that hinders students of hypnosis for conversation from achieving success in establishing rapport is:

They're Trying To Hard!

You cannot force friendship and you cannot force rapport.

It is a waste of time trying to block out the natural, subtle process that is taking place in the background.

The act of trying is to begin consciously blocking a subconscious process.

It's similar to trying to make yourself fall asleep and then attempting to make yourself unconscious It doesn't do the trick!

But you can also build an atmosphere of trust - and intentionally create it in most instances.

So, here's my 4 steps to a formula for rapport:

Four Step Rapport Formula Four Step Rapport Formula

1. Go to an Tattoo Parlour!

Okay, maybe it's not literal.

However, you should revisit the first chapter, where I explained how to be a millionaire, billionaire as well as the queen of England.

Remember the three words I advised you to tattoo onto your forehead?

They're 110 percent of the way to build relationship - and putting them to work on your own will place you above most of the population!

This becomes a lot more powerful If You Can Prove That!

Let people know that you are aware of the place they're at, what they want , and most importantly, who they really are.

Make use of words and stories to convey the reality of your story and show that you are the one who gets the message.

This is incredibly powerful because it lets them know how you are part of their world.

Everyone is in their own universe - with their own perception of

the world colored by their own opinions or prejudices, fears, or desires. The world is not in Rapport the same way unless you're both sharing the same experience.

If you are creating changes, the ultimate aim is to bring your followers to be part of your current reality.

Conclusion

The expression "mind over matter' isn't simply a figurative expression. You've probably realized that after having studied and used an extremely effective techniques for your mind. Even though we've come to the final chapter it is not the end of your journey to hypnosis but rather the beginning. There's plenty to learn and explore regarding the art of hypnosis. There are many options you can attain with the power of hypnosis.

I sincerely hope that this book has equipped you with a solid foundation of the fundamental hypnosis techniques and has enticed you enough to carry on your journey. It is just beginning to discover your full potential, not only as a hypnotist but also the things you are able to achieve with this instrument at your disposal. Be aware that mastering hypnosis involves becoming a master of your mind. For the first time you'll be able to conquer those fears that you thought insurmountable. You can now take on the challenge to develop skills and accomplish goals you thought were impossible to achieve. Hypnosis aims to alter your mental model to reflect the way you would like it. It allows you to reshape any external influence that have taken root in your mind, however it is not beneficial to your health. Use this ability to your benefit If you get the chance, utilize the newfound power with others a hand.

I would definitely recommend that you continue studying, retraining and exploring the potential of the hypnosis process. There are a lot of available resources for different levels of expertise. You might want to think about going to a professional hypnosis clinic or find a teacher. Whatever you decide to do from here I wish you the best!

www.ingramcontent.com/pod-product-compliance
Lightning Source LLC
Chambersburg PA
CBHW060333030426
42336CB00011B/1323